7 STEPS TO
Developing good habits

PLAN
specific action

SIMPLE
you can do it

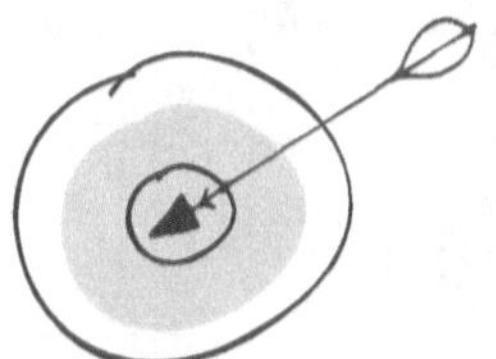

FOCUS
on only one habit at a time

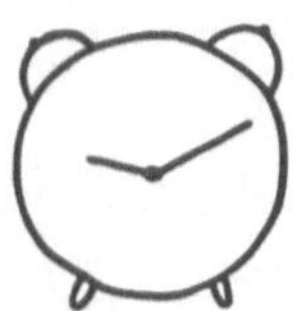

REPEAT
do it everyday

make a social **COMMITMENT**
to perform you habit

REWARD
for every small win

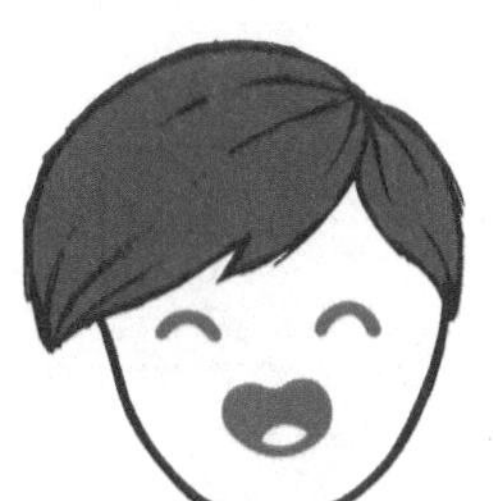

FORGIVE

yourself if you miss a day

My starting point

YOUR PHOTO

	Starting	Goal
Arm		
Chest		
Waist		
Belly		
Hip		
Thigh		
Calf		
Weight		

My Goals :

Cross a big **X** over each day

1	2	3	4	5	6	7	Week 1
8	9	10	11	12	13	14	Week 2
15	16	17	18	19	20	21	Week 3
22	23	24	25	26	27	28	Week 4
29	30	31	32	33	34	35	Week 5
36	37	38	39	40	41	42	Week 6
43	44	45	46	47	48	49	Week 7
50	51	52	53	54	55	56	Week 8
57	58	59	60	61	62	63	Week 9
64	65	66	67	68	69	70	Week 10
71	72	73	74	75	76	77	Week 11
78	79	80	81	82	83	84	Week 12
85	86	87	88	89	90	END	**Win**

Progress Tracker

Day	Arm	Chest	Waist	Belly	Hip	Thigh	Calf	Weight
7								
14								
21								
28								
35								
42								
49								
56								
63								
70								
77								
84								
90								
1								
Different								

You

Can

Do

it

Date: __________________

Su Mo Tu We Th Fr Sa

Fasting Day?   Y   N

8 oz. serving of water

Nutrition

Meals/Snacks/Drinks	Carbs	Fat	Protein	Cals
Total	9	9	9	

Cardio/Strength

Exercises	Set/Reps/Distance	Time

Today I feel / Note :

Date: ___________________   Fasting Day?   Y   N

Su Mo Tu We Th Fr Sa

8 oz. serving of water

Nutrition

Meals/Snacks/Drinks	Carbs	Fat	Protein	Cals
Total	9	9	9	

Cardio/Strength

Exercises	Set/Reps/Distance	Time

Today I feel / Note :

Date: _______________________   **Fasting Day?**   Y   N

Su Mo Tu We Th Fr Sa

Nutrition

8 oz. serving of water

Meals/Snacks/Drinks	Carbs	Fat	Protein	Cals
Total	9	9	9	

Cardio/Strength

Exercises	Set/Reps/Distance	Time

Today I feel / Note :

Date: _________________   Fasting Day?   Y   N

Su Mo Tu We Th Fr Sa

8 oz. serving of water

Nutrition

Meals/Snacks/Drinks	Carbs	Fat	Protein	Cals
Total	9	9	9	

Cardio/Strength

Exercises	Set/Reps/Distance	Time

Today I feel / Note :

Date: ___________________

Su Mo Tu We Th Fr Sa

Fasting Day?   Y   N

8 oz. serving of water

Nutrition

Meals/Snacks/Drinks	Carbs	Fat	Protein	Cals
Total	9	9	9	

Cardio/Strength

Exercises	Set/Reps/Distance	Time

Today I feel / Note :

Date: ....

Su Mo Tu We Th Fr Sa

Fasting Day?   Y   N

8 oz. serving of water

Nutrition

Meals/Snacks/Drinks	Carbs	Fat	Protein	Cals
Total	9	9	9	

Cardio/Strength

Exercises	Set/Reps/Distance	Time

Today I feel / Note :

Date: ....

Su Mo Tu We Th Fr Sa

Fasting Day?   Y   N

8 oz. serving of water

Nutrition

Meals/Snacks/Drinks	Carbs	Fat	Protein	Cals
Total	9	9	9	

Cardio/Strength

Exercises	Set/Reps/Distance	Time

Today I feel / Note :

7

days have passed

YOUR PHOTO

	Day7
Arm	
Chest	
Waist	
Belly	
Hip	
Thigh	
Calf	
Weight	

Thoughts about the week :

....

....

....

Date: _______________   Fasting Day?   Y   N

Su Mo Tu We Th Fr Sa

Nutrition

Meals/Snacks/Drinks	Carbs	Fat	Protein	Cals
Total	9	9	9	

Cardio/Strength

Exercises	Set/Reps/Distance	Time

Today I feel / Note :

Date: _______________________   Fasting Day?   Y   N

Su Mo Tu We Th Fr Sa

                                                 8 oz. serving of water

Nutrition

Meals/Snacks/Drinks	Carbs	Fat	Protein	Cals
Total	9	9	9	

Cardio/Strength

Exercises	Set/Reps/Distance	Time

Today I feel / Note :

Date: ________

Su Mo Tu We Th Fr Sa

Fasting Day?   Y   N

8 oz. serving of water

Nutrition

Meals/Snacks/Drinks	Carbs	Fat	Protein	Cals
Total	g	g	g	

Cardio/Strength

Exercises	Set/Reps/Distance	Time

Today I feel / Note :

Date: ______________   **Fasting Day?**   Y   N

Su Mo Tu We Th Fr Sa

8 oz. serving of water

Nutrition

Meals/Snacks/Drinks	Carbs	Fat	Protein	Cals
Total	9	9	9	

Cardio/Strength

Exercises	Set/Reps/Distance	Time

Today I feel / Note :

Date: _______________

Su Mo Tu We Th Fr Sa

Fasting Day?   Y   N

8 oz. serving of water

Nutrition

Meals/Snacks/Drinks	Carbs	Fat	Protein	Cals
Total	9	9	9	

Cardio/Strength

Exercises	Set/Reps/Distance	Time

Today I feel / Note :

Date: ....   Fasting Day?   Y   N

Su Mo Tu We Th Fr Sa

8 oz. serving of water

Nutrition

Meals/Snacks/Drinks	Carbs	Fat	Protein	Cals
Total	9	9	9	

Cardio/Strength

Exercises	Set/Reps/Distance	Time

Today I feel / Note :

Date: ____________ Fasting Day? Y   N

Su Mo Tu We Th Fr Sa

8 oz. serving of water

Nutrition

Meals/Snacks/Drinks	Carbs	Fat	Protein	Cals
Total	9	9	9	

Cardio/Strength

Exercises	Set/Reps/Distance	Time

Today I feel / Note :

14

days have passed

YOUR PHOTO

	Day 14
Arm	
Chest	
Waist	
Belly	
Hip	
Thigh	
Calf	
Weight	

Thoughts about the week :

....

....

....

Date: ____________________

Su Mo Tu We Th Fr Sa

Fasting Day?   Y   N

8 oz. serving of water

Nutrition

Meals/Snacks/Drinks	Carbs	Fat	Protein	Cals
Total	9	9	9	

Cardio/Strength

Exercises	Set/Reps/Distance	Time

Today I feel / Note :

Date: _______________

Fasting Day?   Y   N

Su Mo Tu We Th Fr Sa

8 oz. serving of water

Nutrition

Meals/Snacks/Drinks	Carbs	Fat	Protein	Cals
Total	9	9	9	

Cardio/Strength

Exercises	Set/Reps/Distance	Time

Today I feel / Note :

Date: ______________   Fasting Day?   Y   N

Su Mo Tu We Th Fr Sa

Nutrition

8 oz. serving of water

Meals/Snacks/Drinks	Carbs	Fat	Protein	Cals
Total	9	9	9	

Cardio/Strength

Exercises	Set/Reps/Distance	Time

Today I feel / Note :

Date: ___________________   Fasting Day?   Y   N

Su Mo Tu We Th Fr Sa

8 oz. serving of water

Nutrition

Meals/Snacks/Drinks	Carbs	Fat	Protein	Cals
Total	9	9	9	

Cardio/Strength

Exercises	Set/Reps/Distance	Time

Today I feel / Note :

Date: _______________

Su Mo Tu We Th Fr Sa

Fasting Day?   Y   N

8 oz. serving of water

Nutrition

Meals/Snacks/Drinks	Carbs	Fat	Protein	Cals
Total	9	9	9	

Cardio/Strength

Exercises	Set/Reps/Distance	Time

Today I feel / Note :

Date: ....

Su Mo Tu We Th Fr Sa

Fasting Day?   Y   N

8 oz. serving of water

Nutrition

Meals/Snacks/Drinks	Carbs	Fat	Protein	Cals
Total	9	9	9	

Cardio/Strength

Exercises	Set/Reps/Distance	Time

Today I feel / Note :

Date: ________________

Su Mo Tu We Th Fr Sa

Fasting Day?   Y   N

8 oz. serving of water

Nutrition

Meals/Snacks/Drinks	Carbs	Fat	Protein	Cals
Total	9	9	9	

Cardio/Strength

Exercises	Set/Reps/Distance	Time

Today I feel / Note :

21
days have passed

YOUR PHOTO

	Day21
Arm	
Chest	
Waist	
Belly	
Hip	
Thigh	
Calf	
Weight	

Thoughts about the week :

Date: _______________

Su Mo Tu We Th Fr Sa

Fasting Day?   Y   N

8 oz. serving of water

Nutrition

Meals/Snacks/Drinks	Carbs	Fat	Protein	Cals
Total	9	9	9	

Cardio/Strength

Exercises	Set/Reps/Distance	Time

Today I feel / Note :

Date: ....   Fasting Day?   Y   N

Su Mo Tu We Th Fr Sa

8 oz. serving of water

Nutrition

Meals/Snacks/Drinks	Carbs	Fat	Protein	Cals
Total	9	9	9	

Cardio/Strength

Exercises	Set/Reps/Distance	Time

Today I feel / Note :

Date: _______________________   Fasting Day?   Y   N

Su Mo Tu We Th Fr Sa

8 oz. serving of water

Nutrition

Meals/Snacks/Drinks	Carbs	Fat	Protein	Cals
Total	9	9	9	

Cardio/Strength

Exercises	Set/Reps/Distance	Time

Today I feel / Note :

Date: ________________

Su Mo Tu We Th Fr Sa

Fasting Day?   Y   N

8 oz. serving of water

Nutrition

Meals/Snacks/Drinks	Carbs	Fat	Protein	Cals
Total	9	9	9	

Cardio/Strength

Exercises	Set/Reps/Distance	Time

Today I feel / Note :

Date: _______________

Su Mo Tu We Th Fr Sa

Nutrition

Fasting Day?   Y   N

8 oz. serving of water

Meals/Snacks/Drinks	Carbs	Fat	Protein	Cals
Total	9	9	9	

Cardio/Strength

Exercises	Set/Reps/Distance	Time

Today I feel / Note :

Date: ______________

Su Mo Tu We Th Fr Sa

Fasting Day?   Y   N

8 oz. serving of water

Nutrition

Meals/Snacks/Drinks	Carbs	Fat	Protein	Cals
Total	9	9	9	

Cardio/Strength

Exercises	Set/Reps/Distance	Time

Today I feel / Note :

Date: ___________________

Su Mo Tu We Th Fr Sa

Fasting Day?   Y   N

8 oz. serving of water

Nutrition

Meals/Snacks/Drinks	Carbs	Fat	Protein	Cals
Total	9	9	9	

Cardio/Strength

Exercises	Set/Reps/Distance	Time

Today I feel / Note :

28
days have passed

YOUR PHOTO

	Day28
Arm	
Chest	
Waist	
Belly	
Hip	
Thigh	
Calf	
Weight	

Thoughts about the week :

Date: _______________

Su Mo Tu We Th Fr Sa

Fasting Day?   Y   N

8 oz. serving of water

Nutrition

Meals/Snacks/Drinks	Carbs	Fat	Protein	Cals
Total	9	9	9	

Cardio/Strength

Exercises	Set/Reps/Distance	Time

Today I feel / Note :

Date: ....

Su Mo Tu We Th Fr Sa

Fasting Day?   Y   N

8 oz. serving of water

Nutrition

Meals/Snacks/Drinks	Carbs	Fat	Protein	Cals
Total	9	9	9	

Cardio/Strength

Exercises	Set/Reps/Distance	Time

Today I feel / Note :

Date: _______________

Fasting Day?   Y   N

Su Mo Tu We Th Fr Sa

8 oz. serving of water

Nutrition

Meals/Snacks/Drinks	Carbs	Fat	Protein	Cals
Total	9	9	9	

Cardio/Strength

Exercises	Set/Reps/Distance	Time

Today I feel / Note :

Date: _______________

Su Mo Tu We Th Fr Sa

Fasting Day?   Y   N

8 oz. serving of water

Nutrition

Meals/Snacks/Drinks	Carbs	Fat	Protein	Cals
Total	9	9	9	

Cardio/Strength

Exercises	Set/Reps/Distance	Time

Today I feel / Note :

Date: _______________

Su Mo Tu We Th Fr Sa

Fasting Day?   Y   N

8 oz. serving of water

Nutrition

Meals/Snacks/Drinks	Carbs	Fat	Protein	Cals
Total	g	g	g	

Cardio/Strength

Exercises	Set/Reps/Distance	Time

Today I feel / Note :

Date: ....   **Fasting Day?**   Y   N

Su Mo Tu We Th Fr Sa

8 oz. serving of water

Nutrition

Meals/Snacks/Drinks	Carbs	Fat	Protein	Cals
Total	9	9	9	

Cardio/Strength

Exercises	Set/Reps/Distance	Time

Today I feel / Note :

Date: ________________

Su Mo Tu We Th Fr Sa

Fasting Day?   Y   N

8 oz. serving of water

Nutrition

Meals/Snacks/Drinks	Carbs	Fat	Protein	Cals
Total	9	9	9	

Cardio/Strength

Exercises	Set/Reps/Distance	Time

Today I feel / Note :

35
days have passed

	Day35
Arm	
Chest	
Waist	
Belly	
Hip	
Thigh	
Calf	
Weight	

Thoughts about the week :

....

....

....

....

Date: ....

Su Mo Tu We Th Fr Sa

Fasting Day?   Y   N

8 oz. serving of water

Nutrition

Meals/Snacks/Drinks	Carbs	Fat	Protein	Cals
Total	9	9	9	

Cardio/Strength

Exercises	Set/Reps/Distance	Time

Today I feel / Note :

Date: ___________

Fasting Day?   Y   N

Su Mo Tu We Th Fr Sa

8 oz. serving of water

Nutrition

Meals/Snacks/Drinks	Carbs	Fat	Protein	Cals
Total	9	9	9	

Cardio/Strength

Exercises	Set/Reps/Distance	Time

Today I feel / Note :

Date: _______________

Su Mo Tu We Th Fr Sa

Fasting Day?   Y   N

8 oz. serving of water

Nutrition

Meals/Snacks/Drinks	Carbs	Fat	Protein	Cals
Total	9	9	9	

Cardio/Strength

Exercises	Set/Reps/Distance	Time

Today I feel / Note :

Date: .... Fasting Day?   Y   N

Su Mo Tu We Th Fr Sa

8 oz. serving of water

Nutrition

Meals/Snacks/Drinks	Carbs	Fat	Protein	Cals
Total	9	9	9	

Cardio/Strength

Exercises	Set/Reps/Distance	Time

Today I feel / Note :

Date: _______________   Fasting Day?   Y   N

Su Mo Tu We Th Fr Sa

8 oz. serving of water

Nutrition

Meals/Snacks/Drinks	Carbs	Fat	Protein	Cals
Total	9	9	9	

Cardio/Strength

Exercises	Set/Reps/Distance	Time

Today I feel / Note :

Date: _______________   **Fasting Day?**   Y   N

Su Mo Tu We Th Fr Sa

8 oz. serving of water

Nutrition

Meals/Snacks/Drinks	Carbs	Fat	Protein	Cals
Total	9	9	9	

Cardio/Strength

Exercises	Set/Reps/Distance	Time

Today I feel / Note :

Date: _______________

Su Mo Tu We Th Fr Sa

Fasting Day?   Y   N

8 oz. serving of water

Nutrition

Meals/Snacks/Drinks	Carbs	Fat	Protein	Cals
Total	g	g	g	

Cardio/Strength

Exercises	Set/Reps/Distance	Time

Today I feel / Note :

42

days have passed

YOUR PHOTO

	Day42
Arm	
Chest	
Waist	
Belly	
Hip	
Thigh	
Calf	
Weight	

Thoughts about the week :

....

....

....

Date: ....

Su Mo Tu We Th Fr Sa

Fasting Day? Y N

Nutrition

8 oz. serving of water

Meals/Snacks/Drinks	Carbs	Fat	Protein	Cals
Total	g	g	g	

Cardio/Strength

Exercises	Set/Reps/Distance	Time

Today I feel / Note :

Date: ....

Su Mo Tu We Th Fr Sa

Fasting Day?   Y   N

8 oz. serving of water

Nutrition

Meals/Snacks/Drinks	Carbs	Fat	Protein	Cals
Total	9	9	9	

Cardio/Strength

Exercises	Set/Reps/Distance	Time

Today I feel / Note :

Date: _______________

Su Mo Tu We Th Fr Sa

Fasting Day?   Y   N

8 oz. serving of water

Nutrition

Meals/Snacks/Drinks	Carbs	Fat	Protein	Cals
Total	9	9	9	

Cardio/Strength

Exercises	Set/Reps/Distance	Time

Today I feel / Note :

Date: ....   Fasting Day?   Y   N

Su Mo Tu We Th Fr Sa

8 oz. serving of water

Nutrition

Meals/Snacks/Drinks	Carbs	Fat	Protein	Cals
Total	9	9	9	

Cardio/Strength

Exercises	Set/Reps/Distance	Time

Today I feel / Note :

Date: _______________

Su Mo Tu We Th Fr Sa

Fasting Day?   Y   N

8 oz. serving of water

Nutrition

Meals/Snacks/Drinks	Carbs	Fat	Protein	Cals
Total	9	9	9	

Cardio/Strength

Exercises	Set/Reps/Distance	Time

Today I feel / Note :

Date: .... Fasting Day?   Y   N

Su Mo Tu We Th Fr Sa

8 oz. serving of water

Nutrition

Meals/Snacks/Drinks	Carbs	Fat	Protein	Cals
Total	9	9	9	

Cardio/Strength

Exercises	Set/Reps/Distance	Time

Today I feel / Note :

Date: ....

Fasting Day?   Y   N

Su Mo Tu We Th Fr Sa

8 oz. serving of water

Nutrition

Meals/Snacks/Drinks	Carbs	Fat	Protein	Cals
Total	9	9	9	

Cardio/Strength

Exercises	Set/Reps/Distance	Time

Today I feel / Note :

49
days have passed

	Day49
Arm	
Chest	
Waist	
Belly	
Hip	
Thigh	
Calf	
Weight	

Thoughts about the week :

....

....

....

Date: ....

Su Mo Tu We Th Fr Sa

Fasting Day?   Y   N

8 oz. serving of water

Nutrition

Meals/Snacks/Drinks	Carbs	Fat	Protein	Cals
Total	9	9	9	

Cardio/Strength

Exercises	Set/Reps/Distance	Time

Today I feel / Note :

Date: ....

Su Mo Tu We Th Fr Sa

Fasting Day?   Y   N

8 oz. serving of water

Nutrition

Meals/Snacks/Drinks	Carbs	Fat	Protein	Cals
Total	9	9	9	

Cardio/Strength

Exercises	Set/Reps/Distance	Time

Today I feel / Note :

Date: ____________

Su Mo Tu We Th Fr Sa

Fasting Day?   Y   N

8 oz. serving of water

Nutrition

Meals/Snacks/Drinks	Carbs	Fat	Protein	Cals
Total	9	9	9	

Cardio/Strength

Exercises	Set/Reps/Distance	Time

Today I feel / Note :

Date: ....

Su Mo Tu We Th Fr Sa

Fasting Day?   Y   N

8 oz. serving of water

Nutrition

Meals/Snacks/Drinks	Carbs	Fat	Protein	Cals
Total	g	g	g	

Cardio/Strength

Exercises	Set/Reps/Distance	Time

Today I feel / Note :

Date: ________________

Su Mo Tu We Th Fr Sa

Fasting Day?   Y   N

8 oz. serving of water

Nutrition

Meals/Snacks/Drinks	Carbs	Fat	Protein	Cals
Total	9	9	9	

Cardio/Strength

Exercises	Set/Reps/Distance	Time

Today I feel / Note :

Date: ....

Su Mo Tu We Th Fr Sa

Fasting Day?   Y   N

8 oz. serving of water

Nutrition

Meals/Snacks/Drinks	Carbs	Fat	Protein	Cals
Total	9	9	9	

Cardio/Strength

Exercises	Set/Reps/Distance	Time

Today I feel / Note :

Date: _______________________

Fasting Day?   Y   N

Su Mo Tu We Th Fr Sa

8 oz. serving of water

Nutrition

Meals/Snacks/Drinks	Carbs	Fat	Protein	Cals
Total	9	9	9	

Cardio/Strength

Exercises	Set/Reps/Distance	Time

Today I feel / Note :

56
days have passed

YOUR PHOTO

	Day56
Arm	
Chest	
Waist	
Belly	
Hip	
Thigh	
Calf	
Weight	

Thoughts about the week :

....

....

....

Date: _______________   Fasting Day?   Y   N

Su Mo Tu We Th Fr Sa

8 oz. serving of water

Nutrition

Meals/Snacks/Drinks	Carbs	Fat	Protein	Cals
Total	g	g	g	

Cardio/Strength

Exercises	Set/Reps/Distance	Time

Today I feel / Note :

Date: .... Fasting Day? Y N

Su Mo Tu We Th Fr Sa

8 oz. serving of water

Nutrition

Meals/Snacks/Drinks	Carbs	Fat	Protein	Cals
Total	9	9	9	

Cardio/Strength

Exercises	Set/Reps/Distance	Time

Today I feel / Note :

Date: ______________

Su Mo Tu We Th Fr Sa

Fasting Day?   Y   N

8 oz. serving of water

Nutrition

Meals/Snacks/Drinks	Carbs	Fat	Protein	Cals
Total	9	9	9	

Cardio/Strength

Exercises	Set/Reps/Distance	Time

Today I feel / Note :

Date: ....   Fasting Day?   Y   N

Su Mo Tu We Th Fr Sa

8 oz. serving of water

Nutrition

Meals/Snacks/Drinks	Carbs	Fat	Protein	Cals
Total	9	9	9	

Cardio/Strength

Exercises	Set/Reps/Distance	Time

Today I feel / Note :

Date: _______________   Fasting Day?   Y   N

Su Mo Tu We Th Fr Sa

8 oz. serving of water

Nutrition

Meals/Snacks/Drinks	Carbs	Fat	Protein	Cals
Total	9	9	9	

Cardio/Strength

Exercises	Set/Reps/Distance	Time

Today I feel / Note :

Date: ....

Su Mo Tu We Th Fr Sa

Fasting Day?   Y   N

8 oz. serving of water

Nutrition

Meals/Snacks/Drinks	Carbs	Fat	Protein	Cals
Total	9	9	9	

Cardio/Strength

Exercises	Set/Reps/Distance	Time

Today I feel / Note :

Date: _______________   Fasting Day?   Y   N

Su Mo Tu We Th Fr Sa

8 oz. serving of water

Nutrition

Meals/Snacks/Drinks	Carbs	Fat	Protein	Cals
Total	g	g	g	

Cardio/Strength

Exercises	Set/Reps/Distance	Time

Today I feel / Note :

63
days have passed

YOUR PHOTO

	Day63
Arm	
Chest	
Waist	
Belly	
Hip	
Thigh	
Calf	
Weight	

Thoughts about the week :

Date: ....

Su Mo Tu We Th Fr Sa

Fasting Day?   Y   N

8 oz. serving of water

Nutrition

Meals/Snacks/Drinks	Carbs	Fat	Protein	Cals
Total	9	9	9	

Cardio/Strength

Exercises	Set/Reps/Distance	Time

Today I feel / Note :

Date: ______________

Su Mo Tu We Th Fr Sa

Fasting Day?   Y   N

8 oz. serving of water

Nutrition

Meals/Snacks/Drinks	Carbs	Fat	Protein	Cals
Total	9	9	9	

Cardio/Strength

Exercises	Set/Reps/Distance	Time

Today I feel / Note :

Date: _______________________   Fasting Day?   Y   N

Su Mo Tu We Th Fr Sa

8 oz. serving of water

Nutrition

Meals/Snacks/Drinks	Carbs	Fat	Protein	Cals
Total	9	9	9	

Cardio/Strength

Exercises	Set/Reps/Distance	Time

Today I feel / Note :

Date: ____________________

Fasting Day?   Y   N

Su Mo Tu We Th Fr Sa

8 oz. serving of water

Nutrition

Meals/Snacks/Drinks	Carbs	Fat	Protein	Cals
Total	9	9	9	

Cardio/Strength

Exercises	Set/Reps/Distance	Time

Today I feel / Note :

Date: ....   Fasting Day?   Y   N

Su Mo Tu We Th Fr Sa

Nutrition

8 oz. serving of water

Meals/Snacks/Drinks	Carbs	Fat	Protein	Cals
Total	g	g	g	

Cardio/Strength

Exercises	Set/Reps/Distance	Time

Today I feel / Note :

Date: ....

Su Mo Tu We Th Fr Sa

Fasting Day?   Y   N

8 oz. serving of water

Nutrition

Meals/Snacks/Drinks	Carbs	Fat	Protein	Cals
Total	9	9	9	

Cardio/Strength

Exercises	Set/Reps/Distance	Time

Today I feel / Note :

Date: ....

Su Mo Tu We Th Fr Sa

Fasting Day?   Y   N

8 oz. serving of water

Nutrition

Meals/Snacks/Drinks	Carbs	Fat	Protein	Cals
Total	9	9	9	

Cardio/Strength

Exercises	Set/Reps/Distance	Time

Today I feel / Note :

70
days have passed

YOUR PHOTO

	Day70
Arm	
Chest	
Waist	
Belly	
Hip	
Thigh	
Calf	
Weight	

Thoughts about the week :

Date: ______________

Su Mo Tu We Th Fr Sa

Fasting Day?   Y   N

8 oz. serving of water

Nutrition

Meals/Snacks/Drinks	Carbs	Fat	Protein	Cals
Total	9	9	9	

Cardio/Strength

Exercises	Set/Reps/Distance	Time

Today I feel / Note :

Date: _______________

Su Mo Tu We Th Fr Sa

Fasting Day?   Y   N

8 oz. serving of water

Nutrition

Meals/Snacks/Drinks	Carbs	Fat	Protein	Cals
Total	9	9	9	

Cardio/Strength

Exercises	Set/Reps/Distance	Time

Today I feel / Note :

Date: _______________

Su Mo Tu We Th Fr Sa

Fasting Day?   Y   N

8 oz. serving of water

Nutrition

Meals/Snacks/Drinks	Carbs	Fat	Protein	Cals
Total	9	9	9	

Cardio/Strength

Exercises	Set/Reps/Distance	Time

Today I feel / Note :

Date: ________________

Su Mo Tu We Th Fr Sa

Fasting Day?   Y   N

8 oz. serving of water

Nutrition

Meals/Snacks/Drinks	Carbs	Fat	Protein	Cals
Total	9	9	9	

Cardio/Strength

Exercises	Set/Reps/Distance	Time

Today I feel / Note :

Date: ....

Su Mo Tu We Th Fr Sa

Fasting Day?   Y   N

8 oz. serving of water

Nutrition

Meals/Snacks/Drinks	Carbs	Fat	Protein	Cals
Total	9	9	9	

Cardio/Strength

Exercises	Set/Reps/Distance	Time

Today I feel / Note :

Date: ....

Su Mo Tu We Th Fr Sa

Fasting Day?   Y   N

8 oz. serving of water

Nutrition

Meals/Snacks/Drinks	Carbs	Fat	Protein	Cals
Total	9	9	9	

Cardio/Strength

Exercises	Set/Reps/Distance	Time

Today I feel / Note :

Date: ____________________   Fasting Day?   Y   N

Su Mo Tu We Th Fr Sa

Nutrition

8 oz. serving of water

Meals/Snacks/Drinks	Carbs	Fat	Protein	Cals
Total	9	9	9	

Cardio/Strength

Exercises	Set/Reps/Distance	Time

Today I feel / Note :

77

days have passed

YOUR PHOTO

	Day77
Arm	
Chest	
Waist	
Belly	
Hip	
Thigh	
Calf	
Weight	

Thoughts about the week :

....

....

....

....

Date: ....

Su Mo Tu We Th Fr Sa

Fasting Day?   Y   N

8 oz. serving of water

Nutrition

Meals/Snacks/Drinks	Carbs	Fat	Protein	Cals
Total	9	9	9	

Cardio/Strength

Exercises	Set/Reps/Distance	Time

Today I feel / Note :

Date: ____________________

Su Mo Tu We Th Fr Sa

Fasting Day?   Y   N

8 oz. serving of water

Nutrition

Meals/Snacks/Drinks	Carbs	Fat	Protein	Cals
Total	9	9	9	

Cardio/Strength

Exercises	Set/Reps/Distance	Time

Today I feel / Note :

Date: _______________   **Fasting Day?**   Y   N

Su Mo Tu We Th Fr Sa

Nutrition

8 oz. serving of water

Meals/Snacks/Drinks	Carbs	Fat	Protein	Cals
Total	9	9	9	

Cardio/Strength

Exercises	Set/Reps/Distance	Time

Today I feel / Note :

Date: ....

Su Mo Tu We Th Fr Sa

Fasting Day?   Y   N

8 oz. serving of water

Nutrition

Meals/Snacks/Drinks	Carbs	Fat	Protein	Cals
Total	9	9	9	

Cardio/Strength

Exercises	Set/Reps/Distance	Time

Today I feel / Note :

Date: ....

Su Mo Tu We Th Fr Sa

Fasting Day?   Y   N

8 oz. serving of water

Nutrition

Meals/Snacks/Drinks	Carbs	Fat	Protein	Cals
Total	9	9	9	

Cardio/Strength

Exercises	Set/Reps/Distance	Time

Today I feel / Note :

Date: ______________   Fasting Day?   Y   N

Su Mo Tu We Th Fr Sa

8 oz. serving of water

Nutrition

Meals/Snacks/Drinks	Carbs	Fat	Protein	Cals
Total	g	g	g	

Cardio/Strength

Exercises	Set/Reps/Distance	Time

Today I feel / Note :

Date: ____________

Fasting Day?   Y   N

Su Mo Tu We Th Fr Sa

Nutrition

8 oz. serving of water

Meals/Snacks/Drinks	Carbs	Fat	Protein	Cals
Total	g	g	g	

Cardio/Strength

Exercises	Set/Reps/Distance	Time

Today I feel / Note :

84
days have passed

YOUR PHOTO

	Day84
Arm	
Chest	
Waist	
Belly	
Hip	
Thigh	
Calf	
Weight	

Thoughts about the week :

Date: ____________________   # Fasting Day?   Y   N

Su Mo Tu We Th Fr Sa

8 oz. serving of water

Nutrition

Meals/Snacks/Drinks	Carbs	Fat	Protein	Cals
Total	9	9	9	

Cardio/Strength

Exercises	Set/Reps/Distance	Time

Today I feel / Note :

Date: ....

Su Mo Tu We Th Fr Sa

Fasting Day?   Y   N

8 oz. serving of water

Nutrition

Meals/Snacks/Drinks	Carbs	Fat	Protein	Cals
Total	9	9	9	

Cardio/Strength

Exercises	Set/Reps/Distance	Time

Today I feel / Note :

Date: _______________   **Fasting Day?**   Y   N

Su Mo Tu We Th Fr Sa

8 oz. serving of water

Nutrition

Meals/Snacks/Drinks	Carbs	Fat	Protein	Cals
Total	9	9	9	

Cardio/Strength

Exercises	Set/Reps/Distance	Time

Today I feel / Note :

Date: ....

Su Mo Tu We Th Fr Sa

Fasting Day?   Y   N

8 oz. serving of water

Nutrition

Meals/Snacks/Drinks	Carbs	Fat	Protein	Cals
Total	9	9	9	

Cardio/Strength

Exercises	Set/Reps/Distance	Time

Today I feel / Note :

Date: .... Fasting Day?   Y   N

Su Mo Tu We Th Fr Sa

8 oz. serving of water

Nutrition

Meals/Snacks/Drinks	Carbs	Fat	Protein	Cals
Total	g	g	g	

Cardio/Strength

Exercises	Set/Reps/Distance	Time

Today I feel / Note :

Date: ....

Su Mo Tu We Th Fr Sa

Nutrition

Fasting Day?   Y   N

8 oz. serving of water

Meals/Snacks/Drinks	Carbs	Fat	Protein	Cals
Total	9	9	9	

Cardio/Strength

Exercises	Set/Reps/Distance	Time

Today I feel / Note :

My Results

	Starting	Day90
Arm		
Chest		
Waist		
Belly		
Hip		
Thigh		
Calf		
Weight		

YOUR PHOTO

My New Goals :

Food Description and Portion Size	Cals (kcal)	Protein (g)	Fat (g)	Carb (g)
100% NATURAL CEREAL 1 OZ	135	3	6	18
1000 ISLAND; SALAD DRSNG;LOCAL 1 TBSP	25	0	2	2
40% BRAN FLAKES; KELLOGG'S 1 OZ	90	4	1	22
ALFALFA SEEDS; SPROUTED; RAW 1 CUP	10	1	0	1
ALL-BRAN CEREAL 1 OZ	70	4	1	21
ALMONDS; WHOLE 1 OZ	165	6	15	6
APPLE JUICE; CANNED 1 CUP	115	0	0	29
APPLE PIE 1 PIECE	405	3	18	60
APPLES; DRIED; SULFURED 10 RINGS	155	1	0	42
APPLES; RAW; PEELED; SLICED 1 CUP	65	0	0	16
APPLES; RAW; UNPEELED;3 PER LB 1 APPLE	80	0	0	21
APPLESAUCE; CANNED; SWEETENED 1 CUP	195	0	0	51
APPLESAUCE; CANNED;UNSWEETENED 1 CUP	105	0	0	28
APRICOT NECTAR; NO ADDED VIT C 1 CUP	140	1	0	36
APRICOT; CANNED; HEAVY SYRUP 1 CUP	215	1	0	55
APRICOTS; CANNED; JUICE PACK 1 CUP	120	2	0	31
APRICOTS; DRIED; COOKED;UNSWTN 1 CUP	210	3	0	55
APRICOTS; DRIED; UNCOOKED 1 CUP	310	5	1	80
APRICOTS; RAW 3 APRCOT	50	1	0	12
ARTICHOKES; GLOBE; COOKED; DRN 1 ARTCHK	55	3	0	12
ASPARAGUS; CKD FRM FRZ;DR;SPER 4 SPEARS	15	2	0	3
ASPARAGUS; CKD FRM FRZ;DRN;CUT 1 CUP	50	5	1	9
ASPARAGUS; CKD FRM RAW; DR;CUT 1 CUP	45	5	1	8
ASPARAGUS;CANNED;SPEARS;W/SALT 4 SPEARS	10	1	0	2
AVOCADOS; CALIFORNIA 1 AVOCDO	305	4	30	12
BAGELS; EGG 1 BAGEL	200	7	2	38
BAGELS; PLAIN 1 BAGEL	200	7	2	38
BAKING POWDER; LOW SODIUM 1 TSP	5	0	0	1
BAKING POWDER;SAS;CAPO4+CASO4 1 TSP	5	0	0	1
BAKING PWDR BISCUITS;FROM MIX 1 BISCUT	95	2	3	14
BAKING PWDR BISCUITS;REFRGDOGH 1 BISCUT	65	1	2	10
BAMBOO SHOOTS; CANNED; DRAINED 1 CUP	25	2	1	4
BANANAS 1 BANANA	105	1	1	27
BANANAS; SLICED 1 CUP	140	2	1	35
BARBECUE SAUCE 1 TBSP	10	0	0	2
BEAN SPROUTS; MUNG; COOKD;DRAN 1 CUP	25	3	0	5
BEAN SPROUTS; MUNG; RAW 1 CUP	30	3	0	6
BEAN WITH BACON SOUP; CANNED 1 CUP	170	8	6	23
BEANS;DRY;CANNED;W/PORK+SWTSCE 1 CUP	385	16	12	54
BEANS;DRY;CANNED;W/PORK+TOMSCE 1 CUP	310	16	7	48
BEEF AND VEGETABLE STEW;HM RCP 1 CUP	220	16	11	15
BEEF BROTH; BOULLN; CONSM;CNND 1 CUP	15	3	1	0
BEEF GRAVY; CANNED 1 CUP	125	9	5	11
BEEF HEART; BRAISED 3 OZ	150	24	5	0
BEEF LIVER; FRIED 3 OZ	185	23	7	7
BEEF NOODLE SOUP; CANNED 1 CUP	85	5	3	9
BEEF POTPIE; HOME RECIPE 1 PIECE	515	21	30	39
BEEF ROAST; EYE O RND; LEAN 2.6 OZ	135	22	5	0
BEEF ROAST; EYE O RND;LEAN+FAT 3 OZ	205	23	12	0
BEEF ROAST; RIB; LEAN + FAT 3 OZ	315	19	26	0
BEEF ROAST; RIB; LEAN ONLY 2.2 OZ	150	17	9	0
BEEF STEAK;SIRLOIN;BROIL;LEAN 2.5 OZ	150	22	6	0
BEEF STEAK;SIRLOIN;BROIL;LN+FT 3 OZ	240	23	15	0
BEEF; CANNED; CORNED 3 OZ	185	22	10	0
BEEF; CKD;BTTM ROUND;LEAN ONLY 2.8 OZ	175	25	8	0
BEEF; CKD;BTTM ROUND;LEAN+ FAT 3 OZ	220	25	13	0
BEEF; CKD;CHUCK BLADE;LEAN+FAT 3 OZ	325	22	26	0
BEEF; CKD;CHUCK BLADE;LEANONLY 2.2 OZ	170	19	9	0
BEEF; DRIED; CHIPPED 2.5 OZ	145	24	4	0
BEER; LIGHT 12 FL OZ	95	1	0	5
BEER; REGULAR 12 FL OZ	150	1	0	13
BEET GREENS; COOKED; DRAINED 1 CUP	40	4	0	8

Food	Cal	Prot	Fat	Carb
BEETS; COOKED; DRAINED; DICED 1 CUP	55	2	0	11
BEETS; COOKED; DRAINED; WHOLE 2 BEETS	30	1	0	7
BLACK BEANS; DRY; COOKED;DRAND1 CUP	225	15	1	41
BLACKEYE PEAS; IMMATR;RAW;CKED1 CUP	180	13	1	30
BLACKEYE PEAS;IMMTR;FRZN;CKED 1 CUP	225	14	1	40
BLACK-EYED PEAS; DRY; COOKED 1 CUP	190	13	1	35
BLUE CHEESE 1 OZ	100	6	8	1
BLUE CHEESE SALAD DRESSING 1 TBSP	75	1	8	1
BLUEBERRIES; FROZEN; SWEETENED1 CUP	185	1	0	50
BLUEBERRIES; FROZEN; SWEETENED10 OZ	230	1	0	62
BOLOGNA 2 SLICES	180	7	16	2
BOSTON BROWN BREAD;W/WHTECRNM 1 SLICE	95	2	1	21
BOSTON BROWN BREAD;W/YLLWCRNML1 SLICE	95	2	1	21
BOUILLON; DEHYDRTD; UNPREPARED1 PKT	15	1	1	1
BRAN MUFFINS; FROM COMMERL MIX1 MUFFIN	140	3	4	24
BRAN MUFFINS; HOME RECIPE 1 MUFFIN	125	3	6	19
BRAUNSCHWEIGER 2 SLICES	205	8	18	2
BRAZIL NUTS 1 OZ	185	4	19	4
BREAD STUFFING;FROM MX;MOIST 1 CUP	420	9	26	40
BREADCRUMBS; DRY; GRATED 1 CUP	390	13	5	73
BROCCOLI; FRZN; COOKED; DRANED1 CUP	50	6	0	10
BROCCOLI; FRZN; COOKED; DRANED1 PIECE	10	1	0	2
BROCCOLI; RAW 1 SPEAR	40	4	1	8
BROWN AND SERVE SAUSAGE;BRWND 1 LINK	50	2	5	0
BROWN GRAVY FROM DRY MIX 1 CUP	80	3	2	14
BROWNIES W/ NUTS;FRM HOME RECP1 BROWNE	95	1	6	11
BROWNIES W/ NUTS;FRSTNG;CMMRCL1 BROWNE	100	1	4	16
BRUSSELS SPROUTS; FRZN; COOKED1 CUP	65	6	1	13
BRUSSELS SPROUTS; RAW; COOKED 1 CUP	60	4	1	13
BUCKWHEAT FLOUR; LIGHT; SIFTED1 CUP	340	6	1	78
BULGUR; UNCOOKED 1 CUP	600	19	3	129
BUTTER; SALTED 1 PAT	35	0	4	0
BUTTER; UNSALTED 1 PAT	35	0	4	0
BUTTER; UNSALTED 1 TBSP	100	0	11	0
BUTTER; UNSALTED 1/2 CUP	810	1	92	0
BUTTERMILK; DRIED 1 CUP	465	41	7	59
BUTTERMILK; FLUID 1 CUP	100	8	2	12
CABBAGE; CHINESE; PAK-CHOI;CKD1 CUP	20	3	0	3
CABBAGE; CHINESE;PE-TSAI; RAW 1 CUP	10	1	0	2
CABBAGE; COMMON; COOKED; DRNED1 CUP	30	1	0	7
CABBAGE; COMMON; RAW 1 CUP	15	1	0	4
CABBAGE; RED; RAW 1 CUP	20	1	0	4
CABBAGE; SAVOY; RAW 1 CUP	20	1	0	4
CAKE OR PASTRY FLOUR; SIFTED 1 CUP	350	7	1	76
CAMEMBERT CHEESE 1 WEDGE	115	8	9	0
CANTALOUP; RAW 1/2 MELN	95	2	1	22
CAP'N CRUNCH CEREAL 1 OZ	120	1	3	23
CARAMELS; PLAIN OR CHOCOLATE 1 OZ	115	1	3	22
CAROB FLOUR 1 CUP	255	6	0	126
CARROT CAKE;CREMCHESE FRST;REC1 PIECE	385	4	21	48
CARROTS; CANNED; DRN; W/ SALT 1 CUP	35	1	0	8
CARROTS; CANNED;DRND; W/O SALT1 CUP	35	1	0	8
CARROTS; COOKED FROM FROZEN 1 CUP	55	2	0	12
CARROTS; COOKED FROM RAW 1 CUP	70	2	0	16
CARROTS; RAW; GRATED 1 CUP	45	1	0	11
CARROTS; RAW; WHOLE 1 CARROT	30	1	0	7
CASHEW NUTS; DRY ROASTD;SALTED1 OZ	165	4	13	9
CASHEW NUTS; DRY ROASTD;UNSALT1 OZ	165	4	13	9
CASHEW NUTS; OIL ROASTD;SALTED1 OZ	165	5	14	8
CASHEW NUTS; OIL ROASTD;UNSALT1 OZ	165	5	14	8
CATSUP 1 CUP	290	5	1	69
CATSUP 1 TBSP	15	0	0	4
CAULIFLOWER; COOKED FROM FROZN1 CUP	35	3	0	7
CAULIFLOWER; COOKED FROM RAW 1 CUP	30	2	0	6

Food	Cal	Prot	Fat	Carb
CAULIFLOWER; RAW 1 CUP	25	2	0	5
CELERY SEED 1 TSP	10	0	1	1
CELERY; PASCAL TYPE; RAW;PIECE1 CUP	20	1	0	4
CELERY; PASCAL TYPE; RAW;STALK1 STALK	5	0	0	1
CHEDDAR CHEESE 1 CU IN	70	4	6	0
CHEDDAR CHEESE 1 OZ	115	7	9	0
CHEERIOS CEREAL 1 OZ	110	4	2	20
CHEESE CRACKERS; PLAIN 10 CRACK	50	1	3	6
CHEESE CRACKERS; SANDWCH;PEANT1 SANDWH	40	1	2	5
CHEESECAKE 1 PIECE	280	5	18	26
CHERRIES; SWEET; RAW 10 CHERY	50	1	1	11
CHERRY PIE 1 PIECE	410	4	18	61
CHESTNUTS; EUROPEAN; ROASTED 1 CUP	350	5	3	76
CHICKEN A LA KING; HOME RECIPE1 CUP	470	27	34	12
CHICKEN CHOW MEIN; CANNED 1 CUP	95	7	0	18
CHICKEN CHOW MEIN; HOME RECIPE1 CUP	255	31	10	10
CHICKEN FRANKFURTER 1 FRANK	115	6	9	3
CHICKEN GRAVY FROM DRY MIX 1 CUP	85	3	2	14
CHICKEN GRAVY; CANNED 1 CUP	190	5	14	13
CHICKEN LIVER; COOKED 1 LIVER	30	5	1	0
CHICKEN NOODLE SOUP; CANNED 1 CUP	75	4	2	9
CHICKEN NOODLE SOUP;DEHYD;PRPD1 PKT	40	2	1	6
CHICKEN POTPIE; HOME RECIPE 1 PIECE	545	23	31	42
CHICKEN RICE SOUP; CANNED 1 CUP	60	4	2	7
CHICKEN ROLL; LIGHT 2 SLICES	90	11	4	1
CHICKEN; CANNED; BONELESS 5 OZ	235	31	11	0
CHICKEN; FRIED; BATTER; BREAST4.9 OZ	365	35	18	13
CHICKEN; FRIED; BATTER;DRMSTCK2.5 OZ	195	16	11	6
CHICKEN; FRIED; FLOUR; BREAST 3.5 OZ	220	31	9	2
CHICKEN; FRIED; FLOUR; DRMSTCK1.7 OZ	120	13	7	1
CHICKEN; ROASTED; DRUMSTICK 1.6 OZ	75	12	2	0
CHICKEN; STEWED; LIGHT + DARK 1 CUP	250	38	9	0
CHICKPEAS; COOKED; DRAINED 1 CUP	270	15	4	45
CHILI CON CARNE W/ BEANS; CNND1 CUP	340	19	16	31
CHILI POWDER 1 TSP	10	0	0	1
CHOCOLATE CHIP COOKIES;COMMRCL4 COOKIE	180	2	9	28
CHOCOLATE CHIP COOKIES;HME RCP4 COOKIE	185	2	11	26
CHOCOLATE CHIP COOKIES;REFRIG 4 COOKIE	225	2	11	32
CHOCOLATE MILK; LOWFAT 2% 1 CUP	180	8	5	26
CHOCOLATE MILK; REGULAR 1 CUP	210	8	8	26
CHOCOLATE; BITTER OT BAKING 1 OZ	145	3	15	8
CINNAMON 1 TSP	5	0	0	2
CLAM CHOWDER; MANHATTAN; CANND1 CUP	80	4	2	12
CLAM CHOWDER; NEW ENG; W/ MILK1 CUP	165	9	7	17
CLAMS; CANNED; DRAINED 3 OZ	85	13	2	2
CLAMS; RAW 3 OZ	65	11	1	2
CLUB SODA 12 FL OZ	0	0	0	0
COCA PWDR W/O NOFAT DRYMLK;PRD1 SERVNG	225	9	9	30
COCA PWDR W/O NONFAT DRY MILK 3/4 OZ	75	1	1	19
COCOA PWDR W/ NOFAT DRMLK;PRPD1 SERVNG	100	3	1	22
COCOA PWDR WITH NONFAT DRYMILK1 OZ	100	3	1	22
COCONUT; DRIED; SWEETND;SHREDD1 CUP	470	3	33	44
COCONUT; RAW; PIECE 1 PIECE	160	1	15	7
COCONUT; RAW; SHREDDED 1 CUP	285	3	27	12
COFFEE; BREWED 6 FL OZ	0	0	0	0
COFFEE; INSTANT; PREPARED 6 FL OZ	0	0	0	1
COFFEECAKE; CRUMB; FROM MIX 1 PIECE	230	5	7	38
COLA; DIET; SACCHARIN ONLY 12 FL OZ	0	0	0	0
COLA; REGULAR 12 FL OZ	160	0	0	41
COLLARDS; COOKED FROM FROZEN 1 CUP	60	5	1	12
COLLARDS; COOKED FROM RAW 1 CUP	25	2	0	5
COOKED SALAD DRSSING; HOME RCP1 TBSP	25	1	2	2
CORN CHIPS 1 OZ	155	2	9	16
CORN FLAKES; KELLOGG'S 1 OZ	110	2	0	24

Food	Calories	Protein (g)	Fat (g)	Carb (g)
CORN FLAKES; TOASTIES 1 OZ	110	2	0	24
CORN GRITS; COOKED; INSTANT 1 PKT	80	2	0	18
CORN GRITS;CKD;REG;WHTE;NOSALT 1 CUP	145	3	0	31
CORN GRITS;CKD;REG;YLLW;NOSALT 1 CUP	145	3	0	31
CORN GRITS;CKD;REG;YLLW;W/SALT 1 CUP	145	3	0	31
CORN MUFFINS; FROM COMMERL MIX 1 MUFFIN	145	3	6	22
CORN MUFFINS; HOME RECIPE 1 MUFFIN	145	3	5	21
CORN OIL 1 TBSP	125	0	14	0
CORN; CNND;CRM STL;WHIT;NO SAL 1 CUP	185	4	1	46
CORN; CNND;CRM STL;WHIT;W/SALT 1 CUP	185	4	1	46
CORN; CNND;CRM STL;YLLW;NO SAL 1 CUP	185	4	1	46
CORN; CNND;CRM STL;YLLW;W/SALT 1 CUP	185	4	1	46
CORN; COOKED FRM FROZN; WHITE 1 CUP	135	5	0	34
CORN; COOKED FRM FROZN; WHITE 1 EAR	60	2	0	14
CORN; COOKED FRM FROZN; YELLOW 1 CUP	135	5	0	34
CORN; COOKED FRM FROZN; YELLOW 1 EAR	60	2	0	14
CORN; COOKED FROM RAW; WHITE 1 EAR	85	3	1	19
CORN; COOKED FROM RAW; YELLOW 1 EAR	85	3	1	19
CORN;CNND;WHL KRNL;WHTE;NO SAL 1 CUP	165	5	1	41
CORN;CNND;WHL KRNL;WHTE;W/SALT 1 CUP	165	5	1	41
CORN;CNND;WHL KRNL;YLLW;NO SAL 1 CUP	165	5	1	41
CORN;CNND;WHL KRNL;YLLW;W/SALT 1 CUP	165	5	1	41
CORNMEAL;BOLTED;DRY FORM 1 CUP	440	11	4	91
CORNMEAL;DEGERMED;ENRCHED;COOK 1 CUP	120	3	0	26
CORNMEAL;DEGERMED;ENRICHED;DRY 1 CUP	500	11	2	108
CORNMEAL;WHOLE-GRND;UNBOLT;DRY 1 CUP	435	11	5	90
COTTAGE CHEESE;CREMD;LRGE CURD 1 CUP	235	28	10	6
COTTAGE CHEESE;CREMD;SMLL CURD 1 CUP	215	26	9	6
COTTAGE CHEESE;CREMD;W/FRUIT 1 CUP	280	22	8	30
COTTAGE CHEESE;LOWFAT 2% 1 CUP	205	31	4	8
COTTAGE CHEESE;UNCREAMED 1 CUP	125	25	1	3
CR OF CHICKEN SOUP W/ H20;CNND 1 CUP	115	3	7	9
CR OF CHICKEN SOUP W/ MLK;CNND 1 CUP	190	7	11	15
CR OF MUSHROM SOUP W/ H2O;CNND 1 CUP	130	2	9	9
CR OF MUSHROM SOUP W/ MLK;CNND 1 CUP	205	6	14	15
CRABMEAT; CANNED 1 CUP	135	23	3	1
CRACKED-WHEAT BREAD 1 SLICE	65	2	1	12
CRACKED-WHEAT BREAD; TOASTED 1 SLICE	65	2	1	12
CRANBERRY JUICE COCKTAL W/VITC 1 CUP	145	0	0	38
CRANBERRY SAUCE; CANNED;SWTND 1 CUP	420	1	0	108
CREAM CHEESE 1 OZ	100	2	10	1
CREAM OF WHEAT;CKD;MIX N EAT 1 PKT	100	3	0	21
CREME PIE 1 PIECE	455	3	23	59
CRM WHEAT;CKD; QUICK; NO SALT 1 CUP	140	4	0	29
CRM WHEAT;CKD;QUICK; W/ SALT 1 CUP	140	4	0	29
CRM WHEAT;CKD;REG;INST;NO SALT 1 CUP	140	4	0	29
CRM WHEAT;CKD;REG;INST;W/SALT 1 CUP	140	4	0	29
CROISSANTS 1 CROSST	235	5	12	27
CUCUMBER; W/ PEEL 6 SLICES	5	0	0	1
CURRY POWDER 1 TSP	5	0	0	1
CUSTARD PIE 1 PIECE	330	9	17	36
CUSTARD; BAKED 1 CUP	305	14	15	29
DANDELION GREENS; COOKED; DRND 1 CUP	35	2	1	7
DANISH PASTRY; FRUIT 1 PASTRY	235	4	13	28
DANISH PASTRY; PLAIN; NO NUTS 1 OZ	110	2	6	13
DANISH PASTRY; PLAIN; NO NUTS 1 PASTRY	220	4	12	26
DATES; CHOPPED 1 CUP	490	4	1	131
DEVIL'S FOOD CAKE;CHOCFRST;FMX 1 CUPCAK	120	2	4	20
DEVIL'S FOOD CAKE;CHOCFRST;FMX 1 PIECE	235	3	8	40
DOUGHNUTS; CAKE TYPE; PLAIN 1 DONUT	210	3	12	24
DOUGHNUTS; YEAST-LEAVEND;GLZED 1 DONUT	235	4	13	26
DUCK; ROASTED; FLESH ONLY 1/2 DUCK	445	52	25	0
EGGNOG 1 CUP	340	10	19	34
EGGPLANT; COOKED; STEAMED 1 CUP	25	1	0	6

Food				
EGGS; COOKED; FRIED 1 EGG	90	6	7	1
EGGS; COOKED; HARD-COOKED 1 EGG	75	6	5	1
EGGS; COOKED; POACHED 1 EGG	75	6	5	1
EGGS; COOKED; SCRAMBLED/OMELET 1 EGG	100	7	7	1
EGGS; RAW; WHITE 1 WHITE	15	4	0	0
EGGS; RAW; WHOLE 1 EGG	75	6	5	1
EGGS; RAW; YOLK 1 YOLK	60	3	5	0
ENCHILADA 1 ENCHLD	235	20	16	24
ENDIVE; CURLY; RAW 1 CUP	10	1	0	2
ENG MUFFIN; EGG; CHEESE; BACON 1 SANDWH	360	18	18	31
ENGLISH MUFFINS; PLAIN 1 MUFFIN	140	5	1	27
ENGLISH MUFFINS; PLAIN; TOASTD 1 MUFFIN	140	5	1	27
EVAPORATED MILK; SKIM; CANNED 1 CUP	200	19	1	29
EVAPORATED MILK; WHOLE; CANNED 1 CUP	340	17	19	25
FATS; COOKING/VEGETBL SHORTENG 1 TBSP	115	0	13	0
FETA CHEESE 1 OZ	75	4	6	1
FIG BARS 4 COOKIE	210	2	4	42
FIGS; DRIED 10 FIGS	475	6	2	122
FILBERTS; (HAZELNUTS) CHOPPED 1 OZ	180	4	18	4
FISH SANDWICH; LGE; W/O CHEESE 1 SANDWH	470	18	27	41
FISH SANDWICH; REG; W/ CHEESE 1 SANDWH	420	16	23	39
FISH STICKS; FROZEN; REHEATED 1 STICK	70	6	3	4
FLOUNDER OR SOLE; BAKED; BUTTR 3 OZ	120	16	6	0
FLOUNDER OR SOLE; BAKED; W/O FAT 3 OZ	80	17	1	0
FONDANT; UNCOATED 1 OZ	105	0	0	27
FRANKFURTER; COOKED 1 FRANK	145	5	13	1
FRENCH BREAD 1 SLICE	100	3	1	18
FRENCH OR VIENNA BREAD 1 LOAF	1270	43	18	230
FRENCH SALAD DRESSING; LOCALOR 1 TBSP	25	0	2	2
FRENCH SALAD DRESSING; REGULAR 1 TBSP	85	0	9	1
FRENCH TOAST; HOME RECIPE 1 SLICE	155	6	7	17
FRIED PIE; APPLE 1 PIE	255	2	14	31
FRIED PIE; CHERRY 1 PIE	250	2	14	32
FROOT LOOPS CEREAL 1 OZ	110	2	1	25
FRUIT COCKTAIL; CNND; HEAVYSYRUP 1 CUP	185	1	0	48
FRUIT COCKTAIL; CNND; JUICE PACK 1 CUP	115	1	0	29
FRUIT PUNCH DRINK; CANNED 6 FL OZ	85	0	0	22
FRUITCAKE; DARK; FROM HOMERECIP 1 CAKE	5185	74	228	783
GARLIC POWDER 1 TSP	10	0	0	2
GELATIN DESSERT; PREPARED 1/2 CUP	70	2	0	17
GELATIN; DRY 1 ENVELP	25	6	0	0
GIN; RUM; VODKA; WHISKY 80-PROOF 1.5 F OZ	95	0	0	0
GIN; RUM; VODKA; WHISKY 86-PROOF 1.5 F OZ	105	0	0	0
GIN; RUM; VODKA; WHISKY 90-PROOF 1.5 F OZ	110	0	0	0
GINGER ALE 12 FL OZ	125	0	0	32
GINGERBREAD CAKE; FROM MIX 1 PIECE	175	2	4	32
GOLDEN GRAHAMS CEREAL 1 OZ	110	2	1	24
GRAHAM CRACKER; PLAIN 2 CRACKR	60	1	1	11
GRAPE DRINK; CANNED 6 FL OZ	100	0	0	26
GRAPE JUICE; CANNED 1 CUP	155	1	0	38
GRAPE SODA 12 FL OZ	180	0	0	46
GRAPEFRT JCE; FRZN; CNCN; UNSWTEN 6 FL OZ	300	4	1	72
GRAPEFRT JCE; FRZN; DLTD; UNSWTEN 1 CUP	100	1	0	24
GRAPEFRUIT JUICE; CANNED; SWTND 1 CUP	115	1	0	28
GRAPEFRUIT JUICE; CANNED; UNSWT 1 CUP	95	1	0	22
GRAPEFRUIT JUICE; RAW 1 CUP	95	1	0	23
GRAPEFRUIT; CANNED; SYRUP PACK 1 CUP	150	1	0	39
GRAPEFRUIT; RAW; PINK 1/2 FRUT	40	1	0	10
GRAPEJCE; FRZN; CONCEN; SWTND; W/C 6 FL OZ	385	1	1	96
GRAPEJCE; FRZN; DILUTD; SWTND; W/C 1 CUP	125	0	0	32
GRAPE-NUTS CEREAL 1 OZ	100	3	0	23
GRAPES; EUROPEAN; RAW; THOMPSN 10 GRAPE	35	0	0	9
GRAPES; EUROPEAN; RAW; TOKAY 10 GRAPE	40	0	0	10
GRAVY AND TURKEY; FROZEN 5 OZ	95	8	4	7

Food				
GREAT NORTHN BEANS;DRY;CKD;DRN1 CUP	210	14	1	38
GROUND BEEF; BROILED; LEAN 3 OZ	230	21	16	0
GROUND BEEF; BROILED; REGULAR 3 OZ	245	20	18	0
GUM DROPS 1 OZ	100	0	0	25
HADDOCK; BREADED; FRIED 3 OZ	175	17	9	7
HALF AND HALF; CREAM 1 CUP	315	7	28	10
HALF AND HALF; CREAM 1 TBSP	20	0	2	1
HALIBUT; BROILED; BUTTER;LEMJU3 OZ	140	20	6	0
HAMBURGER; 4OZ PATTY 1 SANDWH	445	25	21	38
HAMBURGER; REGULAR 1 SANDWH	245	12	11	28
HARD CANDY 1 OZ	110	0	0	28
HERRING; PICKLED 3 OZ	190	17	13	0
HOLLANDAISE SCE; W/ H2O;FRM MX1 CUP	240	5	20	14
HONEY 1 TBSP	65	0	0	17
HONEY NUT CHEERIOS CEREAL 1 OZ	105	3	1	23
HONEYDEW MELON; RAW 1/10 MEL	45	1	0	12
ICE CREAM; VANLLA; REGULR 11% 1 CUP	270	5	14	32
ICE CREAM; VANLLA; RICH 16% FT1 CUP	350	4	24	32
ICE CREAM; VANLLA; SOFT SERVE 1 CUP	375	7	23	38
ICE MILK; VANILLA; 4% FAT 1 CUP	185	5	6	29
ICE MILK; VANILLA;SOFTSERV 3% 1 CUP	225	8	5	38
IMITATION CREAMERS; LIQUID FRZ1 TBSP	20	0	1	2
IMITATION CREAMERS; POWDERED 1 TSP	10	0	1	1
IMITATION WHIPPED TOPPING;FRZN1 CUP	240	1	19	17
IMITATION WHIPPED TOPPING;FRZN1 TBSP	15	0	1	1
IMITATN SOUR DRESSING 1 CUP	415	8	39	11
IMITATN WHIPD TOPING;PRESSRZD 1 CUP	185	1	16	11
IMITATN WHIPD TOPING;PWDRD;PRP1 CUP	150	3	10	13
ITALIAN BREAD 1 SLICE	85	3	0	17
ITALIAN SALAD DRESSING;LOCALOR1 TBSP	5	0	0	2
ITALIAN SALAD DRESSING;REGULAR1 TBSP	80	0	9	1
JAMS AND PRESERVES 1 PKT	40	0	0	10
JAMS AND PRESERVES 1 TBSP	55	0	0	14
JELLIES 1 PKT	40	0	0	10
JELLIES 1 TBSP	50	0	0	13
JELLY BEANS 1 OZ	105	0	0	26
JERUSALEM-ARTICHOKE; RAW 1 CUP	115	3	0	26
KALE; COOKED FROM FROZEN 1 CUP	40	4	1	7
KALE; COOKED FROM RAW 1 CUP	40	2	1	7
KIWIFRUIT; RAW 1 KIWI	45	1	0	11
LAMB; RIB; ROASTED; LEAN + FAT3 OZ	315	18	26	0
LAMB; RIB; ROASTED; LEAN ONLY 2 OZ	130	15	7	0
LAMB;CHOPS;ARM;BRAISED;LEAN 1.7 OZ	135	17	7	0
LAMB;CHOPS;ARM;BRAISED;LEAN+FT2.2 OZ	220	20	15	0
LAMB;CHOPS;LOIN;BROIL;LEAN 2.3 OZ	140	19	6	0
LAMB;CHOPS;LOIN;BROIL;LEAN+FAT2.8 OZ	235	22	16	0
LAMB;LEG;ROASTED; LEAN ONLY 2.6 OZ	140	20	6	0
LARD 1 TBSP	115	0	13	0
LEMON JUICE; CANNED 1 CUP	50	1	1	16
LEMON JUICE; CANNED 1 TBSP	5	0	0	1
LEMON JUICE; RAW 1 CUP	60	1	0	21
LEMON JUICE;FRZN;SINGLE-STRNGH6 FL OZ	55	1	1	16
LEMON MERINGUE PIE 1 PIE	2140	31	86	317
LEMON MERINGUE PIE 1 PIECE	355	5	14	53
LEMONADE;CONCEN;FRZEN;DILUTED 6 FL OZ	80	0	0	21
LEMON-LIME SODA 12 FL OZ	155	0	0	39
LEMONS; RAW 1 LEMON	15	1	0	5
LENTILS; DRY; COOKED 1 CUP	215	16	1	38
LETTUCE; BUTTERHEAD; RAW;HEAD 1 HEAD	20	2	0	4
LETTUCE; BUTTERHEAD; RAW;LEAVE1 LEAF	0	0	0	0
LETTUCE; CRISPHEAD; RAW; HEAD 1 HEAD	70	5	1	11
LETTUCE; CRISPHEAD; RAW;PIECES1 CUP	5	1	0	1
LETTUCE; CRISPHEAD; RAW;WEDGE 1 WEDGE	20	1	0	3
LETTUCE; LOOSELEAF 1 CUP	10	1	0	2

Food	Cal			
LIGHT; COFFEE OR TABLE CREAM 1 CUP	470	6	46	9
LIGHT; COFFEE OR TABLE CREAM 1 TBSP	30	0	3	1
LIMA BEANS; DRY; COOKED;DRANED 1 CUP	260	16	1	49
LIMA BEANS;BABY; FRZN;CKED;DRN 1 CUP	190	12	1	35
LIMA BEANS;THICK SEED;FRZN;CKD 1 CUP	170	10	1	32
LIME JUICE; RAW 1 CUP	65	1	0	22
LIME JUICE;CANNED 1 CUP	50	1	1	16
LIMEADE;CONCEN;FROZEN;DILUTED 6 FL OZ	75	0	0	20
LIMEADE;CONCENTRATE;FRZN;UNDIL 6 FL OZ	410	0	0	108
LUCKY CHARMS CEREAL 1 OZ	110	3	1	23
MACADAMIA NUTS; OILRSTD;SALTED 1 OZ	205	2	22	4
MACARONI AND CHEESE; CANNED 1 CUP	230	9	10	26
MACARONI AND CHEESE; HOME RCPE 1 CUP	430	17	22	40
MACARONI; COOKED; FIRM 1 CUP	190	7	1	39
MACARONI; COOKED; TENDER; HOT 1 CUP	155	5	1	32
MACARONI; COOKED; TENDER;COLD 1 CUP	115	4	0	24
MALTED MILK; CHOCOLATE; POWDER 3/4 OZ	85	1	1	18
MALTED MILK;CHOCOLATE; PWDRPPD 1 SERVNG	235	9	9	29
MALTED MILK;NATURAL; POWDER 3/4 OZ	85	3	2	15
MALTED MILK;NATURAL; PWDR PPRD 1 SERVNG	235	11	10	27
MALT-O-MEAL; W/O SALT 1 CUP	120	4	0	26
MALT-O-MEAL; WITH SALT 1 CUP	120	4	0	26
MANGOS; RAW 1 MANGO	135	1	1	35
MARGARINE; IMITATION 40% FAT 1 TBSP	50	0	5	0
MARGARINE; IMITATION 40% FAT 8 OZ	785	1	88	1
MARGARINE; REGULR;HARD;80% FAT 1 PAT	35	0	4	0
MARGARINE; SPREAD;HARD;60% FAT 1 PAT	25	0	3	0
MARGARINE; SPREAD;HARD;60% FAT 1/2 CUP	610	1	69	0
MARGARINE; SPREAD;SOFT;60% FAT 1 TBSP	75	0	9	0
MARSHMALLOWS 1 OZ	90	1	0	23
MAYONNAISE TYPE SALAD DRESSING 1 TBSP	60	0	5	4
MAYONNAISE; IMITATION 1 TBSP	35	0	3	2
MAYONNAISE; REGULAR 1 TBSP	100	0	11	0
MELBA TOAST; PLAIN 1 PIECE	20	1	0	4
MILK CHOCOLATE CANDY; PLAIN 1 OZ	145	2	9	16
MILK CHOCOLATE CANDY;W/ ALMOND 1 OZ	150	3	10	15
MILK CHOCOLATE CANDY;W/ PENUTS 1 OZ	155	4	11	13
MILK CHOCOLATE CANDY;W/ RICE C 1 OZ	140	2	7	18
MILK; LOFAT; 1%; ADDED SOLIDS 1 CUP	105	9	2	12
MILK; LOFAT; 1%; NO ADDEDSOLID 1 CUP	100	8	3	12
MILK; LOFAT; 2%; ADDED SOLIDS 1 CUP	125	9	5	12
MILK; LOFAT; 2%; NO ADDEDSOLID 1 CUP	120	8	5	12
MILK; SKIM; ADDED MILK SOLIDS 1 CUP	90	9	1	12
MILK; SKIM; NO ADDED MILKSOLID 1 CUP	85	8	0	12
MILK; WHOLE; 3.3% FAT 1 CUP	150	8	8	11
MINESTRONE SOUP; CANNED 1 CUP	80	4	3	11
MISO 1 CUP	470	29	13	65
MIXED GRAIN BREAD 1 SLICE	65	2	1	12
MIXED GRAIN BREAD; TOASTED 1 SLICE	65	2	1	12
MIXED NUTS W/ PEANTS;DRY;SALTD 1 OZ	170	5	15	7
MIXED NUTS W/ PEANTS;DRY;UNSLT 1 OZ	170	5	15	7
MIXED NUTS W/ PEANTS;OIL;SALTD 1 OZ	175	5	16	6
MIXED NUTS W/ PEANTS;OIL;UNSLT 1 OZ	175	5	16	6
MOLASSES; CANE; BLACKSTRAP 2 TBSP	85	0	0	22
MOZZARELLA CHEESE; WHOLE MILK 1 OZ	80	6	6	1
MOZZARELLA CHESE;SKIM; LOMOIST 1 OZ	80	8	5	1
MUENSTER CHEESE 1 OZ	105	7	9	0
MUSHROOM GRAVY; CANNED 1 CUP	120	3	6	13
MUSHROOMS; CANNED; DRND;W/SALT 1 CUP	35	3	0	8
MUSHROOMS; COOKED; DRAINED 1 CUP	40	3	1	8
MUSHROOMS; RAW 1 CUP	20	1	0	3
MUSTARD GREENS; COOKED; DRANED 1 CUP	20	3	0	3
MUSTARD; PREPARED; YELLOW 1 TSP	5	0	0	0
NATURE VALLEY GRANOLA CEREAL 1 OZ	125	3	5	19

Food				
NECTARINES; RAW 1 NECTRN	65	1	1	16
NONFAT DRY MILK; INSTANTIZED 1 CUP	245	24	0	35
NONFAT DRY MILK; INSTANTIZED 1 ENVLPE	325	32	1	47
NOODLES; CHOW MEIN; CANNED 1 CUP	220	6	11	26
NOODLES; EGG; COOKED 1 CUP	200	7	2	37
OATMEAL BREAD 1 SLICE	65	2	1	12
OATMEAL BREAD; TOASTED 1 SLICE	65	2	1	12
OATMEAL W/ RAISINS COOKIES 4 COOKIE	245	3	10	36
OATMEAL;CKD;INSTNT;FLVRD;FORTF 1 PKT	160	5	2	31
OATMEAL;CKD;INSTNT;PLAIN;FORTF 1 PKT	105	4	2	18
OATMEAL;CKD;RG;QCK;INST;W/OSAL 1 CUP	145	6	2	25
OATMEAL;CKD;RG;QCK;INST;W/SALT 1 CUP	145	6	2	25
OCEAN PERCH; BREADED; FRIED 1 FILLET	185	16	11	7
OKRA PODS; COOKED 8 PODS	25	2	0	6
OLIVE OIL 1 TBSP	125	0	14	0
OLIVES; CANNED; GREEN 4 MEDIUM	15	0	2	0
OLIVES; CANNED; RIPE; MISSION 3 SMALL	15	0	2	0
ONION POWDER 1 TSP	5	0	0	2
ONION RINGS; BREADED;FRZN;PRPD 2 RINGS	80	1	5	8
ONIONS; RAW; CHOPPED 1 CUP	55	2	0	12
ONIONS; RAW; COOKED; DRAINED 1 CUP	60	2	0	13
ONIONS; RAW; SLICED 1 CUP	40	1	0	8
ONIONS; SPRING; RAW 6 ONION	10	1	0	2
ORANGE JUICE; CANNED 1 CUP	105	1	0	25
ORANGE JUICE; CHILLED 1 CUP	110	2	1	25
ORANGE JUICE; RAW 1 CUP	110	2	0	26
ORANGE JUICE;FROZEN CONCENTRTE 6 FL OZ	340	5	0	81
ORANGE JUICE;FRZN;CNCN;DILUTED 1 CUP	110	2	0	27
ORANGE SODA 12 FL OZ	180	0	0	46
ORANGES; RAW 1 ORANGE	60	1	0	15
ORANGES; RAW; SECTIONS 1 CUP	85	2	0	21
OREGANO 1 TSP	5	0	0	1
OYSTERS; BREADED; FRIED 1 OYSTER	90	5	5	5
OYSTERS; RAW 1 CUP	160	20	4	8
PANCAKES; BUCKWHEAT; FROM MIX 1 PANCAK	55	2	2	6
PANCAKES; PLAIN; FROM MIX 1 PANCAK	60	2	2	8
PANCAKES; PLAIN; HOME RECIPE 1 PANCAK	60	2	2	9
PAPAYAS; RAW 1 CUP	65	1	0	17
PAPRIKA 1 TSP	5	0	0	1
PARMESAN CHEESE; GRATED 1 CUP	455	42	30	4
PARMESAN CHEESE; GRATED 1 OZ	130	12	9	1
PARMESAN CHEESE; GRATED 1 TBSP	25	2	2	0
PARSLEY; FREEZE-DRIED 1 TBSP	0	0	0	0
PARSLEY; RAW 10 SPRIG	5	0	0	1
PARSNIPS; COOKED; DRAINED 1 CUP	125	2	0	30
PASTERZD PROCES CHEESE; SWISS 1 OZ	95	7	7	1
PASTERZD PROCES CHEESE;AMERICN 1 OZ	105	6	9	0
PASTERZD PROCES CHESE FOOD;AMR 1 OZ	95	6	7	2
PASTERZD PROCES CHESE SPRED;AM 1 OZ	80	5	6	2
PEA BEANS; DRY; COOKED;DRAINED 1 CUP	225	15	1	40
PEA; GREEN; SOUP; CANNED 1 CUP	165	9	3	27
PEACH PIE 1 PIECE	405	4	17	60
PEACHES; CANNED; HEAVY SYRUP 1 CUP	190	1	0	51
PEACHES; CANNED; HEAVY SYRUP 1 HALF	60	0	0	16
PEACHES; CANNED; JUICE PACK 1 CUP	110	2	0	29
PEACHES; CANNED; JUICE PACK 1 HALF	35	0	0	9
PEACHES; DRIED;COOKED;UNSWETND 1 CUP	200	3	1	51
PEACHES; FROZEN;SWETNED;W/VITC 1 CUP	235	2	0	60
PEACHES; FROZEN;SWETNED;W/VITC 10 OZ	265	2	0	68
PEACHES; RAW 1 PEACH	35	1	0	10
PEACHES; RAW; SLICED 1 CUP	75	1	0	19
PEANUT BUTTER 1 TBSP	95	5	8	3
PEANUT BUTTER COOKIE;HOME RECP 4 COOKIE	245	4	14	28
PEANUT OIL 1 CUP	1910	0	216	0

PEANUT OIL 1 TBSP	125	0	14	0
PEANUTS; OIL ROASTED; SALTED 1 OZ	165	8	14	5
PEANUTS; OIL ROASTED; UNSALTED1 CUP	840	39	71	27
PEANUTS; OIL ROASTED; UNSALTED1 OZ	165	8	14	5
PEARS; CANNED; HEAVY SYRUP 1 CUP	190	1	0	49
PEARS; CANNED; HEAVY SYRUP 1 HALF	60	0	0	15
PEARS; CANNED; JUICE PACK 1 CUP	125	1	0	32
PEARS; CANNED; JUICE PACK 1 HALF	40	0	0	10
PEARS; RAW; BARTLETT 1 PEAR	100	1	1	25
PEARS; RAW; BOSC 1 PEAR	85	1	1	21
PEARS; RAW; D'ANJOU 1 PEAR	120	1	1	30
PEAS; EDIBLE POD; COOKED;DRNED1 CUP	65	5	0	11
PEAS; GREEN;CNND;DRND; W/ SALT1 CUP	115	8	1	21
PEAS; GREEN;CNND;DRND;W/O SALT1 CUP	115	8	1	21
PEAS; SPLIT; DRY; COOKED 1 CUP	230	16	1	42
PEAS;GRN; FROZEN COOKED;DRANED1 CUP	125	8	0	23
PECAN PIE 1 PIECE	575	7	32	71
PECANS; HALVES 1 CUP	720	8	73	20
PECANS; HALVES 1 OZ	190	2	19	5
PEPPER; BLACK 1 TSP	5	0	0	1
PEPPERS; HOT CHILI; RAW; GREEN1 PEPPER	20	1	0	4
PEPPERS; HOT CHILI; RAW; RED 1 PEPPER	20	1	0	4
PEPPERS; SWEET; COOKED; GREEN 1 PEPPER	15	0	0	3
PEPPERS; SWEET; COOKED; RED 1 PEPPER	15	0	0	3
PEPPERS; SWEET; RAW; GREEN 1 PEPPER	20	1	0	4
PEPPERS; SWEET; RAW; RED 1 PEPPER	20	1	0	4
PEPPER-TYPE SODA 12 FL OZ	160	0	0	41
PICKLES; CUCUMBER; DILL 1 PICKLE	5	0	0	1
PICKLES; CUCUMBER; FRESH PACK 2 SLICES	10	0	0	3
PICKLES; CUCUMBER; SWT GHERKIN1 PICKLE	20	0	0	5
PINE NUTS 1 OZ	160	3	17	5
PINEAPPLE JUICE; CANNED;UNSWTN1 CUP	140	1	0	34
PINEAPPLE; CANNED; HEAVY SYRUP1 CUP	200	1	0	52
PINEAPPLE; CANNED; HEAVY SYRUP1 SLICE	45	0	0	12
PINEAPPLE; CANNED; JUICE PACK 1 CUP	150	1	0	39
PINEAPPLE; CANNED; JUICE PACK 1 SLICE	35	0	0	9
PINEAPPLE; RAW; DICED 1 CUP	75	1	1	19
PINEAPPLE-GRAPEFRUIT JUICEDRNK6 FL OZ	90	0	0	23
PINTO BEANS;DRY;COOKED;DRAINED1 CUP	265	15	1	49
PISTACHIO NUTS 1 OZ	165	6	14	7
PITA BREAD 1 PITA	165	6	1	33
PIZZA; CHEESE 1 SLICE	290	15	9	39
PLANTAINS; COOKED 1 CUP	180	1	0	48
PLANTAINS; RAW 1 PLANTN	220	2	1	57
PLUMS; CANNED; HEAVY SYRUP 1 CUP	230	1	0	60
PLUMS; CANNED; HEAVY SYRUP 3 PLUMS	120	0	0	31
PLUMS; CANNED; JUICE PACK 1 CUP	145	1	0	38
PLUMS; CANNED; JUICE PACK 3 PLUMS	55	0	0	14
PLUMS; RAW; 1-1/2-IN DIAM 1 PLUM	15	0	0	4
PLUMS; RAW; 2-1/8-IN DIAM 1 PLUM	35	1	0	9
POPCORN; AIR-POPPED; UNSALTED 1 CUP	30	1	0	6
POPCORN; POPPED; VEG OIL;SALTD1 CUP	55	1	3	6
POPCORN; SUGAR SYRUP COATED 1 CUP	135	2	1	30
POPSICLE 1 POPCLE	70	0	0	18
PORK CHOP; LOIN; BROIL; LEAN 2.5 OZ	165	23	8	0
PORK CHOP; LOIN; BROIL; LEN+FT3.1 OZ	275	24	19	0
PORK CHOP; LOIN;PANFRY; LEAN 2.4 OZ	180	19	11	0
PORK CHOP; LOIN;PANFRY;LEAN+FT3.1 OZ	335	21	27	0
PORK FRESH HAM; ROASTD; LEAN 2.5 OZ	160	20	8	0
PORK FRESH HAM; ROASTD;LEAN+FT3 OZ	250	21	18	0
PORK FRESH RIB; ROASTD; LEAN 2.5 OZ	175	20	10	0
PORK FRESH RIB; ROASTD;LEAN+FT3 OZ	270	21	20	0
PORK SHOULDER; BRAISD; LEAN 2.4 OZ	165	22	8	0
PORK SHOULDER; BRAISD;LEAN+FAT3 OZ	295	23	22	0

PORK; CURED; BACON; REGUL;CKED 3 SLICE	110	6	9	0
PORK; CURED; BACON;CANADN;CKED 2 SLICE	85	11	4	1
PORK; CURED; HAM; CANNED;ROAST 3 OZ	140	18	7	0
PORK; CURED; HAM; ROSTED;LEAN 2.4 OZ	105	17	4	0
PORK; CURED; HAM; ROSTED;LN+FT 3 OZ	205	18	14	0
PORK; LINK; COOKED 1 LINK	50	3	4	0
PORK; LUNCHEON MEAT;CANNED 2 SLICES	140	5	13	1
PORK; LUNCHEON MEAT;CHOPPD HAM 2 SLICES	95	7	7	0
PORK; LUNCHEON MEAT;CKD HAM;LN 2 SLICES	75	11	3	1
PORK; LUNCHEON MEAT;CKD HAM;RG 2 SLICES	105	10	6	2
POTATO CHIPS 10 CHIPS	105	1	7	10
POTATO SALAD MADE W/ MAYONNAIS 1 CUP	360	7	21	28
POTATOES; AU GRATIN; FROM MIX 1 CUP	230	6	10	31
POTATOES; AU GRATIN; HOME RECP 1 CUP	325	12	19	28
POTATOES; BAKED FLESH ONLY 1 POTATO	145	3	0	34
POTATOES; BAKED WITH SKIN 1 POTATO	220	5	0	51
POTATOES; BOILED; PEELED AFTER 1 POTATO	120	3	0	27
POTATOES; BOILED; PEELED BEFOR 1 POTATO	115	2	0	27
POTATOES; HASHED BROWN;FR FRZN 1 CUP	340	5	18	44
POTATOES; MASHED;FRM DEHYDRTED 1 CUP	235	4	12	32
POTATOES; MASHED;RECPE;MLK+MAR 1 CUP	225	4	9	35
POTATOES; MASHED;RECPE;W/ MILK 1 CUP	160	4	1	37
POTATOES; SCALLOPED; FROM MIX 1 CUP	230	5	11	31
POTATOES; SCALLOPED; HOME RECP 1 CUP	210	7	9	26
POTATOES;FRENCH-FRD;FRZN;FRIED 10 STRIP	160	2	8	20
POTATOES;FRENCH-FRD;FRZN;OVEN 10 STRIP	110	2	4	17
POUND CAKE; FROM HOME RECIPE 1 SLICE	120	2	5	15
PRETZELS; STICK 10 PRETZ	10	0	0	2
PRETZELS; TWISTED; DUTCH 1 PRETZ	65	2	1	13
PRETZELS; TWISTED; THIN 10 PRETZ	240	6	2	48
PRODUCT 19 CEREAL 1 OZ	110	3	0	24
PROVOLONE CHEESE 1 OZ	100	7	8	1
PRUNE JUICE; CANNED 1 CUP	180	2	0	45
PRUNES; DRIED 5 LARGE	115	1	0	31
PRUNES; DRIED; COOKED;UNSWTNED 1 CUP	225	2	0	60
PUDDING; CHOC; COOKED FROM MIX 1/2 CUP	150	4	4	25
PUDDING; CHOC; INSTANT; FR MIX 1/2 CUP	155	4	4	27
PUDDING; CHOCOLATE;CANNED 5 OZ	205	3	11	30
PUDDING; RICE; FROM MIX 1/2 CUP	155	4	4	27
PUDDING; TAPIOCA; CANNED 5 OZ	160	3	5	28
PUDDING; TAPIOCA; FROM MIX 1/2 CUP	145	4	4	25
PUDDING; VANILLA; CANNED 5 OZ	220	2	10	33
PUDDING; VNLLA;COOKED FROM MIX 1/2 CUP	145	4	4	25
PUDDING; VNLLA;INSTANT FRM MIX 1/2 CUP	150	4	4	27
PUMPERNICKEL BREAD 1 SLICE	80	3	1	16
PUMPERNICKEL BREAD; TOASTED 1 SLICE	80	3	1	16
PUMPKIN AND SQUASH KERNELS 1 OZ	155	7	13	5
PUMPKIN PIE 1 PIECE	320	6	17	37
PUMPKIN; CANNED 1 CUP	85	3	1	20
PUMPKIN; COOKED FROM RAW 1 CUP	50	2	0	12
QUICHE LORRAINE 1 SLICE	600	13	48	29
RADISHES; RAW 4 RADISH	5	0	0	1
RAISIN BRAN; KELLOGG'S 1 OZ	90	3	1	21
RAISIN BRAN; POST 1 OZ	85	3	1	21
RAISIN BREAD 1 SLICE	65	2	1	13
RAISIN BREAD; TOASTED 1 SLICE	65	2	1	13
RAISINS 1 CUP	435	5	1	115
RAISINS 1 PACKET	40	0	0	11
RASPBERRIES; FROZEN; SWEETENED 1 CUP	255	2	0	65
RASPBERRIES; FROZEN; SWEETENED 10 OZ	295	2	0	74
RASPBERRIES; RAW 1 CUP	60	1	1	14
RED KIDNEY BEANS; DRY; CANNED 1 CUP	230	15	1	42
REFRIED BEANS; CANNED 1 CUP	295	18	3	51
RELISH; SWEET 1 TBSP	20	0	0	5

Food				
RHUBARB; COOKED; ADDED SUGAR 1 CUP	280	1	0	75
RICE KRISPIES CEREAL 1 OZ	110	2	0	25
RICE; BROWN; COOKED 1 CUP	230	5	1	50
RICE; WHITE; COOKED 1 CUP	225	4	0	50
RICE; WHITE; INSTANT; COOKED 1 CUP	180	4	0	40
RICE; WHITE; PARBOILED; COOKED 1 CUP	185	4	0	41
RICE; WHITE; PARBOILED; RAW 1 CUP	685	14	1	150
RICE; WHITE; RAW 1 CUP	670	12	1	149
RICOTTA CHEESE; PART SKIM MILK 1 CUP	340	28	19	13
RICOTTA CHEESE; WHOLE MILK 1 CUP	430	28	32	7
ROAST BEEF SANDWICH 1 SANDWH	345	22	13	34
ROLLS; DINNER; COMMERCIAL 1 ROLL	85	2	2	14
ROLLS; DINNER; HOME RECIPE 1 ROLL	120	3	3	20
ROLLS; FRANKFURTER + HAMBURGER 1 ROLL	115	3	2	20
ROLLS; HARD 1 ROLL	155	5	2	30
ROLLS; HOAGIE OR SUBMARINE 1 ROLL	400	11	8	72
ROOT BEER 12 FL OZ	165	0	0	42
RYE BREAD; LIGHT 1 SLICE	65	2	1	12
RYE BREAD; LIGHT; TOASTED 1 SLICE	65	2	1	12
RYE WAFERS; WHOLE-GRAIN 2 WAFERS	55	1	1	10
SAFFLOWER OIL 1 TBSP	125	0	14	0
SALAMI; COOKED TYPE 2 SLICES	145	8	11	1
SALAMI; DRY TYPE 2 SLICES	85	5	7	1
SALMON; BAKED; RED 3 OZ	140	21	5	0
SALMON; CANNED; PINK; W/ BONES 3 OZ	120	17	5	0
SALMON; SMOKED 3 OZ	150	18	8	0
SALT 1 TSP	0	0	0	0
SALTINES 4 CRACKR	50	1	1	9
SANDWICH SPREAD; PORK; BEEF 1 TBSP	35	1	3	2
SANDWICH TYPE COOKIE 4 COOKIE	195	2	8	29
SARDINES; ATLNTC;CNNED;OIL;DRN 3 OZ	175	20	9	0
SAUERKRAUT; CANNED 1 CUP	45	2	0	10
SCALLOPS; BREADED; FRZN;REHEAT 6 SCALOP	195	15	10	10
SEAWEED; KELP; RAW 1 OZ	10	0	0	3
SEAWEED; SPIRULINA; DRIED 1 OZ	80	16	2	7
SELF-RISING FLOUR; UNSIFTED 1 CUP	440	12	1	93
SEMISWEET CHOCOLATE 1 CUP	860	7	61	97
SESAME SEEDS 1 TBSP	45	2	4	1
SHAKES; THICK; CHOCOLATE 10 OZ	335	9	8	60
SHAKES; THICK; VANILLA 10 OZ	315	11	9	50
SHEETCAKE;W/ WHFRSTNG;HOMERCIP 1 PIECE	445	4	14	77
SHEETCAKE;W/O FRSTNG;HOMERECIP 1 PIECE	315	4	12	48
SHERBET; 2% FAT 1 CUP	270	2	4	59
SHORTBREAD COOKIE; COMMERCIAL 4 COOKIE	155	2	8	20
SHORTBREAD COOKIE; HOME RECIPE 2 COOKIE	145	2	8	17
SHREDDED WHEAT CEREAL 1 OZ	100	3	1	23
SHRIMP; CANNED; DRAINED 3 OZ	100	21	1	1
SHRIMP; FRENCH FRIED 3 OZ	200	16	10	11
SNACK CAKES;DEVILS FOOD;CREMFLSM CAKE	105	1	4	17
SNACK CAKES;SPONGE CREME FLLNGSM CAKE	155	1	5	27
SNACK TYPE CRACKERS 1 CRACKR	15	0	1	2
SNAP BEAN;CNND;DRND;GREEN;SALT 1 CUP	25	2	0	6
SNAP BEAN;CNND;DRND;GRN;NOSALT 1 CUP	25	2	0	6
SNAP BEAN;CNND;DRND;YLLW; SALT 1 CUP	25	2	0	6
SNAP BEAN;CNND;DRND;YLLW;NOSAL 1 CUP	25	2	0	6
SNAP BEAN;FRZ;CKD;DRND;GREEN 1 CUP	35	2	0	8
SNAP BEAN;FRZ;CKD;DRND;YELLOW 1 CUP	35	2	0	8
SNAP BEAN;RAW;CKD;DRND;GREEN 1 CUP	45	2	0	10
SNAP BEAN;RAW;CKD;DRND;YELLOW 1 CUP	45	2	0	10
SOUR CREAM 1 TBSP	25	0	3	1
SOY SAUCE 1 TBSP	10	2	0	2
SOYBEAN OIL; HYDROGENATED 1 TBSP	125	0	14	0
SOYBEAN-COTTONSEED OIL; HYDRGN 1 TBSP	125	0	14	0
SOYBEANS; DRY; COOKED; DRAINED 1 CUP	235	20	10	19

Food				
SPAGHETTI; COOKED; FIRM 1 CUP	190	7	1	39
SPAGHETTI; COOKED; TENDER 1 CUP	155	5	1	32
SPAGHETTI; TOM SAUCE CHEE;HMRP1 CUP	260	9	9	37
SPAGHETTI; TOM SAUCE CHEES;CND1 CUP	190	6	2	39
SPAGHETTI;MEATBALLS;TOMSA;HMRP1 CUP	330	19	12	39
SPAGHETTI;MEATBALLS;TOMSAC;CND1 CUP	260	12	10	29
SPECIAL K CEREAL 1 OZ	110	6	0	21
SPINACH SOUFFLE 1 CUP	220	11	18	3
SPINACH; CANNED; DRND;W/ SALT 1 CUP	50	6	1	7
SPINACH; CANNED; DRND;W/O SALT1 CUP	50	6	1	7
SPINACH; COOKED FR FRZEN; DRND1 CUP	55	6	0	10
SPINACH; COOKED FROM RAW; DRND1 CUP	40	5	0	7
SPINACH; RAW 1 CUP	10	2	0	2
SQUASH; SUMMER; COOKED; DRAIND1 CUP	35	2	1	8
SQUASH; WINTER; BAKED 1 CUP	80	2	1	18
STRAWBERRIES; FROZEN; SWEETEND1 CUP	245	1	0	66
STRAWBERRIES; FROZEN; SWEETEND10 OZ	275	2	0	74
STRAWBERRIES; RAW 1 CUP	45	1	1	10
SUGAR COOKIE; FROM REFRIG DOGH4 COOKIE	235	2	12	31
SUGAR FROSTED FLAKES; KELLOGG 1 OZ	110	1	0	26
SUGAR SMACKS CEREAL 1 OZ	105	2	1	25
SUGAR; BROWN; PRESSED DOWN 1 CUP	820	0	0	212
SUGAR; POWDERED; SIFTED 1 CUP	385	0	0	100
SUGAR; WHITE; GRANULATED 1 PKT	25	0	0	6
SUGAR; WHITE; GRANULATED 1 TBSP	45	0	0	12
SUNFLOWER OIL 1 TBSP	125	0	14	0
SUNFLOWER SEEDS 1 OZ	160	6	14	5
SUPER SUGAR CRISP CEREAL 1 OZ	105	2	0	26
SWEET (DARK) CHOCOLATE 1 OZ	150	1	10	16
SWEETPOTATOES; BAKED; PEELED 1 POTATO	115	2	0	28
SWEETPOTATOES; CANDIED 1 PIECE	145	1	3	29
SWEETPOTATOES; CNNED; VAC PACK1 PIECE	35	1	0	8
SWISS CHEESE 1 OZ	105	8	8	1
SYRUP; CHOCOLATE FLAVORED THIN2 TBSP	85	1	0	22
SYRUP; CHOCOLATE FLVRED; FUDGE2 TBSP	125	2	5	21
TABLE SYRUP (CORN AND MAPLE) 2 TBSP	122	0	0	32
TACO 1 TACO	195	9	11	15
TAHINI 1 TBSP	90	3	8	3
TANGERINE JUICE; CANNED;SWTNED1 CUP	125	1	0	30
TANGERINES; CANNED; LIGHT SYRP1 CUP	155	1	0	41
TANGERINES; RAW 1 TANGRN	35	1	0	9
TARTAR SAUCE 1 TBSP	75	0	8	1
TEA; BREWED 8 FL OZ	0	0	0	0
TEA; INSTANT;PREPRD;UNSWEETEND8 FL OZ	0	0	0	1
TEA;INSTANT;PREPARD;SWEETENED 8 FL OZ	85	0	0	22
TOASTER PASTRIES 1 PASTRY	210	2	6	38
TOFU 1 PIECE	85	9	5	3
TOMATO JUICE; CANNED W/O SALT 1 CUP	40	2	0	10
TOMATO JUICE; CANNED WITH SALT1 CUP	40	2	0	10
TOMATO PASTE; CANNED W/O SALT 1 CUP	220	10	2	49
TOMATO PASTE; CANNED WITH SALT1 CUP	220	10	2	49
TOMATO PUREE; CANNED W/O SALT 1 CUP	105	4	0	25
TOMATO PUREE; CANNED WITH SALT1 CUP	105	4	0	25
TOMATO SOUP W/ WATER; CANNED 1 CUP	85	2	2	17
TOMATO SOUP WITH MILK; CANNED 1 CUP	160	6	6	22
TOMATO VEG SOUP; DEHYD;PREPRED1 PKT	40	1	1	8
TOMATOES; CANNED; S+L; W/ SALT1 CUP	50	2	1	10
TOMATOES; CANNED; S+L;W/O SALT1 CUP	50	2	1	10
TOMATOES; RAW 1 TOMATO	25	1	0	5
TORTILLAS; CORN 1 TORTLA	65	2	1	13
TOTAL CEREAL 1 OZ	100	3	1	22
TRIX CEREAL 1 OZ	110	2	0	25
TROUT; BROILED; W/ BUTTR;LEMJU3 OZ	175	21	9	0
TUNA SALAD 1 CUP	375	33	19	19

Food				
TUNA; CANND; DRND;OIL;CHK;LGHT3 OZ	165	24	7	0
TUNA; CANND; DRND;WATR; WHITE 3 OZ	135	30	1	0
TURKEY HAM; CURED TURKEY THIGH2 SLICES	75	11	3	0
TURKEY LOAF; BREAST MEAT W/O C2 SLICES	45	10	1	0
TURKEY LOAF; BREAST MEAT; W/ C2 SLICES	45	10	1	0
TURKEY PATTIES; BRD;BATTD;FRID1 PATTY	180	9	12	10
TURKEY ROAST; FRZN;LGHT+DRK;CK3 OZ	130	18	5	3
TURKEY; ROASTED; DARK MEAT 4 PIECES	160	24	6	0
TURKEY; ROASTED; LIGHT + DARK 1 CUP	240	41	7	0
TURKEY; ROASTED; LIGHT + DARK 3 PIECES	145	25	4	0
TURKEY; ROASTED; LIGHT MEAT 2 PIECES	135	25	3	0
TURNIP GREENS; CKED FRM FROZEN1 CUP	50	5	1	8
TURNIP GREENS; COOKED FROM RAW1 CUP	30	2	0	6
TURNIPS; COOKED; DICED 1 CUP	30	1	0	8
VANILLA WAFERS 10 COOKE	185	2	7	29
VEAL CUTLET; MED FAT;BRSD;BRLD3 OZ	185	23	9	0
VEAL RIB; MED FAT; ROASTED 3 OZ	230	23	14	0
VEGETABLE BEEF SOUP; CANNED 1 CUP	80	6	2	10
VEGETABLE JUICE COCKTAIL; CNND1 CUP	45	2	0	11
VEGETABLES; MIXED; CANNED 1 CUP	75	4	0	15
VEGETABLES; MIXED; CKED FR FRZ1 CUP	105	5	0	24
VEGETARIAN SOUP; CANNED 1 CUP	70	2	2	12
VIENNA BREAD 1 SLICE	70	2	1	13
VIENNA SAUSAGE 1 SAUSAG	45	2	4	0
VINEGAR AND OIL SALAD DRESSING1 TBSP	70	0	8	0
VINEGAR; CIDER 1 TBSP	0	0	0	1
WAFFLES; FROM HOME RECIPE 1 WAFFLE	245	7	13	26
WAFFLES; FROM MIX 1 WAFFLE	205	7	8	27
WALNUTS; ENGLISH; PIECES 1 CUP	770	17	74	22
WALNUTS; ENGLISH; PIECES 1 OZ	180	4	18	5
WATERMELON; RAW 1 PIECE	155	3	2	35
WATERMELON; RAW; DICED 1 CUP	50	1	1	11
WHEAT BREAD; TOASTED 1 SLICE	65	3	1	12
WHEAT FLOUR; ALL-PURPOSE;SIFTD1 CUP	420	12	1	88
WHEAT FLOUR; ALL-PURPOSE;UNSIF1 CUP	455	13	1	95
WHEAT; THIN CRACKERS 4 CRACKR	35	1	1	5
WHEATIES CEREAL 1 OZ	100	3	0	23
WHIPPED TOPPING; PRESSURIZED 1 CUP	155	2	13	7
WHIPPED TOPPING; PRESSURIZED 1 TBSP	10	0	1	0
WHIPPING CREAM; UNWHIPED;LIGHT1 CUP	700	5	74	7
WHITE BREAD CRUMBS; SOFT 1 CUP	120	4	2	22
WHITE BREAD CUBES 1 CUP	80	2	1	15
WHITE BREAD; SLICE 18 PER LOAF1 SLICE	65	2	1	12
WHITE BREAD; SLICE 22 PER LOAF1 SLICE	55	2	1	10
WHITE BREAD; TOASTED 18 PER 1 SLICE	65	2	1	12
WHITE BREAD; TOASTED 22 PER 1 SLICE	55	2	1	10
WHITE CAKE W/ WHT FRSTNG;COMML1 PIECE	260	3	9	42
WHITE SAUCE W/ MILK FROM MIX 1 CUP	240	10	13	21
WHITE SAUCE; MEDIUM; HOME RECP1 CUP	395	10	30	24
WHOLE-WHEAT BREAD 1 SLICE	70	3	1	13
WHOLE-WHEAT BREAD; TOASTED 1 SLICE	70	3	1	13
WHOLE-WHEAT FLOUR;HRD WHT;STIR1 CUP	400	16	2	85
WHOLE-WHEAT WAFERS; CRACKERS 2 CRACKR	35	1	2	5
WINE; DESSERT 3.5 F OZ	140	0	0	8
WINE; TABLE; RED 3.5 F OZ	75	0	0	3
WINE; TABLE; WHITE 3.5 F OZ	80	0	0	3
YEAST; BAKERS; DRY; ACTIVE 1 PKG	20	3	0	3
YEAST; BREWERS; DRY 1 TBSP	25	3	0	3
YELLOW CAKE W/ CHOC FRST;FRMIX1 PIECE	235	3	8	40
YELLOWCAKE W/ CHOCFRSTNG;COMML1 PIECE	245	2	11	39
YOGURT; W/ LOFAT MILK; PLAIN 8 OZ	145	12	4	16
YOGURT; W/ LOFAT MILK;FRUITFLV8 OZ	230	10	2	43
YOGURT; W/ NONFAT MILK 8 OZ	125	13	0	17
YOGURT; W/ WHOLE MILK 8 OZ	140	8	7	11

www.ingramcontent.com/pod-product-compliance
Lightning Source LLC
Chambersburg PA
CBHW031244250726
48655CB00005B/2074